P9-CBG-344

WITHDRAWN

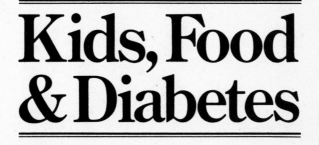

Kids, Food & Diabetes

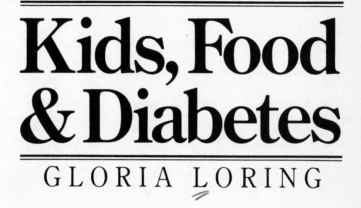

Kids, Food
& Diabetes

GLORIA LORING

CONTEMPORARY
BOOKS, INC.
CHICAGO ■ NEW YORK

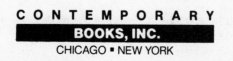
RODMAN PUBLIC LIBRARY

641.563
L873
A-1

Library of Congress Cataloging-in-Publication Data

Loring, Gloria.
   Kids, food, and diabetes: a book of recipes, menus,
   and practical advice.

   Bibliography: p.
   Includes index.
   1. Diabetes in children—Diet therapy.   2. Diabetes
in youth—Diet therapy.   3. Diabetes in children—
Diet therapy—Recipes.   4. Diabetes in youth—Diet
therapy—Recipes.   I. Title.
RJ420.D5L67   1986   641.5'6314'088054   86-16689
ISBN 0-8092-4956-1

Copyright © 1986 by Gloria Loring
All rights reserved
Published by Contemporary Books, Inc.
180 North Michigan Avenue, Chicago, Illinois 60601
Manufactured in the United States of America
Library of Congress Catalog Card Number: 86-16689
International Standard Book Number: 0-8092-4956-1

Published simultaneously in Canada by Beaverbooks, Ltd.
195 Allstate Parkway, Valleywood Business Park
Markham, Ontario L3R 4T8 Canada

Recipes by Jane Brody on pages 94, 102, 134, 167, 172, 216, 260, and 287 from *Jane Brody's Good Food Book: Living the High-Carbohydrate Way* by Jane E. Brody. Reprinted by permission of W. W. Norton & Company, Inc. Copyright © 1985 by Jane E. Brody.

Recipes by Mabel Cavaiani on pages 171, 175, 180, 186, and 292 from *The New Diabetic Cookbook* by Mabel Cavaiani. Reprinted by permission of Contemporary Books, Inc. Copyright © 1984 by Mabel Cavaiani.

Recipes by Katharine Middleton and Mary Abbott Hess on pages 93, 160, 275, 284, and 290 from *The Art of Cooking for the Diabetic* by Katharine Middleton and Mary Abbott Hess. Reprinted by permission of Contemporary Books, Inc. Copyright © 1978 by Katharine Middleton and Mary Abbott Hess.

Peach Whip recipe on page 162 courtesy of Jell-O® Brand Gelatin.

Oat Bran Muffins recipe on page 109 courtesy of the Quaker Oats Company.

This book is dedicated to Donald, who shows me every day, in a hundred small ways, what love is.

Contents

As We Go to Press

As this is being written, the American Diabetes Association and the American Dietetic Association are in the process of slightly revising some of the food exchange values. If you have any questions, make sure to ask your dietitian or physician, or contact your local American Diabetes Association affiliate.

Foreword

My first and only experience cooking for a diabetic was a disaster. As a senior in high school I dated a boy who happened to be diabetic. At Christmastime I got the bright idea to bake for him using a sugar substitute. One slight problem: not knowing any better, and without a diabetic cookbook, I followed the standard cookie recipe to the letter, substituting equal parts Sweet'n Low for sugar. I will never forget the scene that followed. My mother, also a diabetic, volunteered to taste the final product. How she survived the experience I will never know—the expression on her face said it all. The cookies were anything but sweet and didn't exactly melt in your mouth! To be honest, they had the consistency of rubber. The next thing I knew, my sister and a friend were attempting to dribble my creations, warm from the oven, across the kitchen floor. When they asked if we still had a field hockey stick in the garage, I knew my diabetic meal planning days were over.

Luckily, I was not responsible for this boy's nutrition, because I didn't know the first thing about food and diabetes. Since I was a senior in high school, it was a funny situation. Had I been the parent of a newly diagnosed diabetic, it wouldn't have been so funny.

Nutrition is extremely important in treating diabetes. As *Kids, Food, and Diabetes* shows us, it's the quality, as well as the quantity, that counts. The fact of the matter is we would all be much healthier if we ate in moderation, using less salt, less sugar, more fiber, and fresher, more natural foods.

Following a diabetic diet does not have to be torture; instead, with a little planning and invention, it can be medically correct as well as appealing to the entire family. Exchange information, diet planning, and recipes have come a long way in the nine years since my cookie fiasco.

Gloria Loring stresses living with diabetes. She reminds us of the importance of putting child first, diabetic second; kids *are* kids. Kids test themselves and their parents most of the time; kids with diabetes are no different. Ups and downs are to be expected.

For the diabetic and nondiabetic alike, *Kids, Food, and Diabetes* is a great introduction to understanding the many facets of diabetes. It helps to know you're not alone. How lucky we are that Gloria has taken time to share her experiences as a parent of a child with diabetes. She will help all of us live happier, healthier, active lives, accepting and living with diabetes.

Gloria, my personal thanks for *Kids, Food, and Diabetes*, your endless energy, and your determination to do all you can.

Kathryn Iacocca Hentz
President, The Iacocca Foundation*

---

*The Iacocca Foundation was established to fund diabetes research.

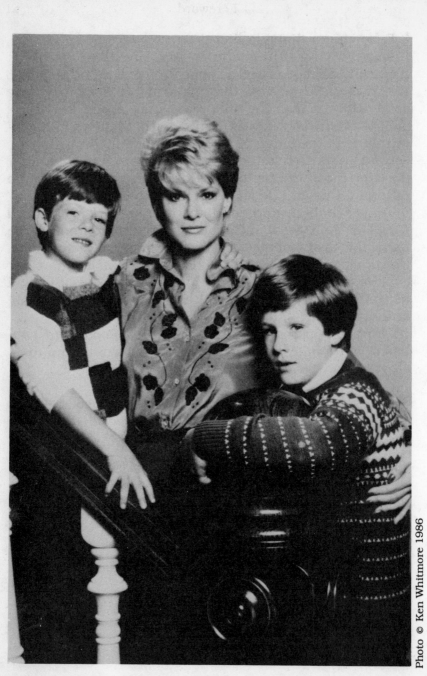

Photo © Ken Whitmore 1986

Gloria Loring with sons Robin (left) and Brennan (right).

Preface

In a sense, this book has been in development for more than seven years. It began the day I learned my son had diabetes. Since then, I have grown from a frightened parent to a confident comanager of my son's diabetes. I have talked with other parents and shared frustrations with them. I have written about diabetes by helping to formulate the storyline and dialogue when my television daughter on "Days of Our Lives" was diagnosed as diabetic. I have given countless interviews to broaden awareness of the disease. I have appeared in concerts to raise money for research. I have lobbied in Congress and hosted telethons. I have produced an album and published cookbooks to keep the researchers in business. I have learned and am still learning. This book is an attempt to share what I know. Thanks to the many health professionals who helped me, I have come to know a lot more through writing it.

It will become clear as you read along that this is not merely another diabetes cookbook. I have been interested in healthful food and good nutrition for 20 years. Good nutrition is more than eating the proper number of calories or exchanges each day. The quality of food is important. In this book, I have stressed using fresh fruits and vegetables, homemade soup stock, and whole grains. The better the quality of ingredients used in a recipe, the better the final result. Fresh, whole foods also offer more nourishment for your body. Many "health-food nuts" have been advocating whole natural foods for a long time. The science of nutrition is now beginning to support what some of us have believed all along. One of my purposes in writing this book was to encourage better nutrition for everyone, not just diabetics.

The book is divided into three sections. Part I is called "Nutrition." It gives you information and, I hope, incentive to feed your family the best possible diet. It discusses the exchange diet and gives basic exchange information in addition to giving you a short course in reading labels and figuring exchanges. There is a chapter on stocking your kitchen with healthy foods and on determining which utensils and gadgets you might find helpful. The last chapter of this section is about special occasions. It gives you ideas about how to handle camping trips, holidays, parties, restaurants, and sporting events. Part II is "The Cookbook." It is divided into four meal chapters, each containing an introduction, which list exchanges for all recipes to assist in overall planning and provide menu ideas and lots of recipes. In the Appendix you'll find a master list of recipes to help you plan your menus.

Part III is called "The Copebook." The first chapter, "Perspective," is meant to serve as an overview of the patterns of child development and how the stages of development relate to diabetes. It offers suggestions for dealing with emotional and psychological problems that may arise.

The next chapter, "Specifics: Questions from Parents," addresses many topics of concern to parents of children with diabetes. It covers, in detail, many of the ramifications of diabetes, from sick-day problems, to insulin reactions, to sibling rivalry and more.

"Resources" offers a partial list of some of the organizations and companies you can turn to for information and support. If you haven't yet done so, you should contact them all and gather as much material as you can to increase your understanding of this disease. There also is a list of some books I feel you might find beneficial.

The final chapter is "Research." Its purpose is to motivate you to join those of us who raise money so that we can end this disease once and for all.

Being a modern woman (I hope), I grappled with the issue of gender usage in this book. I decided to use *he* and *she* alternately so that (whether your child is male or female) you can relate as directly as possible to what I offer.

This book was originally meant to be just a nutrition/recipe book, but as I wrote, I felt the need to share, parent to parent, information I feel may be useful to you. By no means is this book intended to give all the answers or present the only good ways to handle problems that arise. There are many very good books I've listed in "Resources" that deal with the technical aspects of diabetes care in greater depth. Please read them to broaden your knowledge and, of course, always call your health professional if you have questions.

What I've tried most to achieve in writing this book is the creation of a practical, loving volume of support for the difficult task of caring for a diabetic child.

One last thing. If you are interested in obtaining the *Days of Our Lives Celebrity Cookbook*, Volumes I and II, or my album, *A Shot in the Dark*, or if you just want to write, write to me at the address below. All proceeds of the books and record are donated to diabetes research.

Gloria Loring
14755 Ventura Blvd.
Ste. 744
Sherman Oaks, CA 91403

Acknowledgments

I want to give my love and thanks:

To Donald, for reminding me there is enough time and showing me there is always enough love.

To my sons, for being understanding about all the nights Mom had to work on her book.

To Tina, for giving so freely of her time and knowledge.

To Judy, my secretary, assistant, and friend, for handling all areas of my life.

To Patty, for all the hours spent discussing recipes.

To Beth, for great proofreading and for being the best possible friend.

To Peggy, my dear sister, for her support and help.

To Tenley, for flying fingers and enthusiasm.

To Jody Rein, my editor, for being patient and for encouraging a nervous, harried author.

To Lee Ducat and Gloria Pennington, for their shining examples of achievement.

To Karen Hostetler and all the JDF parents who gave their time and love.

And to Drs. Jonathan Kellerman, Robert Clemons, Julio Santiago, and his team members Susan Green Davis, Jeanne Bubb, and Debra Kahn, Sherman Holvey, and researchers Phyllis Crapo and Ronald Kahn, for sharing their expertise with me.

Introduction

Sharing knowledge, experience, and feelings is one of the great gifts that people can give to each other.

Though there is no shortcut for the authenticity of one's personal experience, the comfort and reassurance from knowing that you are not alone and that others have walked the same path is therapeutic.

In talking with and caring for thousands of persons with diabetes and their families over the past thirty years, I have learned that the fears, anxieties, frustrations, and depression associated with the presence of diabetes are significantly relieved by finding out how others cope. Parents in particular are eager to communicate with others and share their experiences.

Every day I am impressed by the willingness of mothers and fathers to devote time and energy to help raise funds for research and to support organizations that serve the cause of diabetes prevention and treatment. Every day I am asked, "What can I do to help?" And every day I am made aware of the continuing need to provide "real world" diabetes education to families and others involved with persons who have diabetes.

Physicians and other health care professionals are working hard to teach the fundamentals of diabetes and to provide the skills necessary to achieve and maintain good health; but the value of exchanging experiences and knowledge between those who must daily face living with diabetes is immeasurable.

Gloria Loring learned firsthand the impact of having a diabetic son. She turned her fears and concerns into a

determination to help obtain money for research to find a
cure for diabetes. In addition, she became acutely aware of
the need parents have for information about diabetes. She
also realized that she could make an important contribu-
tion by informing parents and all individuals who are
interested in diabetes about some of the important les-
sons that she has learned from personal experience.

Ms. Loring is a "master giver." She has drawn from her
own search for information, consulted with experts, and
written what she wanted to know when her son developed
diabetes seven years ago. I am impressed by the quality of
the practical, up-to-date information she provides.
Though *Kids, Food, and Diabetes* is designed to be a
"parent-to-parent" book, its value extends to everyone
who has or is touched by diabetes. From cooking to
coping, it includes basic information about nutrition and
diet, specific meal options, and wonderful recipes incor-
porating the most recent ideas about proper nutritional
provisions. With humor and serious attention to details
about issues that everyone wants (and needs) to know,
Gloria Loring describes her experiences and those of
others, explaining patterns of behavior from infancy to
adolescence and how diabetes has an impact on these
stages. She also deals with parental roles and needs and
provides information about resources available for additional support and help.

I recommend that physicians use this book as a supplement to the education provided in their diabetes teaching
programs. It can help all of you all the days of your lives.

Sherman Holvey, M.D.
Diabetologist and Past
President, American Diabetes
Association of Southern California

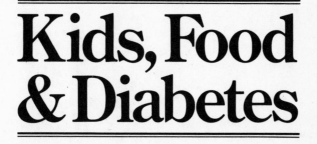

Kids, Food & Diabetes

PART I
NUTRITION

1
The Basics

Children will never eat anything that has not danced on TV.

Erma Bombeck

Having a child with diabetes has brought many changes into your life. Many of them are very difficult, but not all of them are negative. One positive change is an increased awareness of good nutrition.

The changes you make in this area vary depending on your family's dietary habits B.D. (before diabetes). For example, I had always been extremely health-conscious concerning Brennan's diet. In truth, I was called a health-food nut. I breast-fed Brennan for 20 months and made all his baby food from scratch. No sugar- or salt-laden canned baby foods for my son! I kept no candy, soda, or chips in the house. Ice cream and cookies were occasional treats. I allowed Brennan to eat whatever he wanted as long as it was healthful food; if he wanted three oranges for a snack, that was fine with me. When Brennan was diagnosed, that changed. All these rules and restrictions were suddenly placed on us. I had always promised myself I would not nag my children about food. Well, here I was with a child who loved eating, and because of diabetes, food became an issue between us. The timing of meals also became a problem. When Brennan was on one shot, he had to eat by 5:30 or he would have a reaction. That problem was solved when he started two shots a day. We didn't have to give as much NPH in his morning shot, so he "bottomed out" less frequently in the afternoon. At

3

least then we could sit down together and have dinner as a family.

Family support is a vital element in diabetes management. It doesn't mean that no one in the family can ever again eat candy or enjoy a dessert. What is important is that the whole family basically eats the same meals. Besides being good for your diabetic child psychologically, the diabetic diet may be the healthiest thing that ever happened to your family.

There is a vast body of evidence that indicates that the current American diet contains too much fat, sugar, salt, and animal protein and not enough fiber. Studies have linked our diet to increased risk of developing heart disease, cancer, obesity, osteoporosis, and Type II diabetes. The diet you and your family will follow because of diabetes has the same underlying principles as the diet for a healthy heart and the diet recommended by the American Cancer Society.

People like to eat what they're used to eating. That means you may need to adjust your family's diet a little at a time. It also means that you are influencing their eating patterns and their health for the rest of their lives.

This section is designed to inspire you to follow the best principles of nutrition known today. It's much easier to make changes and stick to them when you know why you are doing so. Within that framework, there are special requirements of the diabetic diet that are covered in the chapter on food exchanges and in Part III, "The Copebook."

All of the nutrition information in this book has been written under the guidance of Tina Leeser. Tina earned her bachelor of science degree at the University of Michigan and her master's degree in nutrition at Texas Women's University. She worked with juvenile diabetics at Texas Children's Hospital in Houston for four years. Tina is presently the Diabetes Education Specialist at Cedars-Sinai Medical Center in Beverly Hills. She has personal as well as professional experience with diabetes, and this book could not have been written without her.

FAT

In the average American diet, fat accounts for more than 40 percent of our total calories. Most of the fat we consume is merely empty calories. One tablespoon of vegetable oil a day would satisfy our nutritional requirement. We now consume, on the average, eight times that amount, or the equivalent of one stick of butter per day! In the process, we eat many unnecessary calories. Fat provides two and a quarter times more calories than does protein; there are nine calories per gram of fat compared to four calories per gram of protein. It's even more fattening than alcohol, which has seven calories per gram.

Fat and its partner, cholesterol, are culprits in our two most deadly diseases, heart disease and cancer. Fat is a very real concern for diabetics too, since they have an increased risk of heart disease. It is true that the body manufactures its own cholesterol (serum cholesterol), but it is handled differently from the cholesterol we ingest (dietary cholesterol). Studies indicate that internally manufactured cholesterol results in the manufacture of needed hormones, cell membranes, and protective sheaths for nerve fibers. Dietary cholesterol, however, enters the general circulation and takes a more direct path to blood vessels. Everyone in your family will benefit from a diet lower in fats and cholesterol.

Fats fall into two basic categories: saturated and unsaturated. Saturated fats are solid at room temperature. They increase the amount of cholesterol in the general circulation. Animal fats are highly saturated. Two vegetable fats—palm oil and coconut oil—are also saturated. They're used in processed foods because they're cheap and don't turn rancid easily.

The fats found in fish are oils that are less saturated and, according to recent studies, may be very good for you. Fish oil contains a group of substances called *Omega-3 long-chain fatty acids.* When consumed frequently, they appear to be more effective than polyunsaturated oil in reducing the risk of heart disease. Some heart experts are now urging more frequent consumption of fatty fishes like tuna, sardines, salmon, swordfish, trout, and herring. In addition, squid and shellfish have a high proportion of Omega-3 long-chain fatty acids. Mussels, oysters, scallops, and clams are especially desirable because they are low-cholesterol foods as well.

Shrimp is relatively high in cholesterol compared to other fish (90 milligrams in 3 ounces), but that amount is only one-third of the cholesterol found in one egg yolk. Shellfish is, in general, very low in fat and, therefore, low in calories. The cholesterol in shellfish has a different bond configuration and some experts feel it may not affect serum cholesterol levels in the same way as other animal proteins.

Unsaturated fats, which are oils at room temperature, don't have adverse effects on blood cholesterol. In fact, both polyunsaturates and monounsaturates help lower blood cholesterol. Olive oil and peanut oil are monounsaturates and are the main fats used in Japan, Greece, and Italy, where heart disease rates are very low.

It is not enough merely to switch from butter and lard to oils. We need to decrease the total amount of fats in our daily food intake. Remember, all that is needed per day is one tablespoon of vegetable oil, three FAT exchanges, to fulfill our requirements for essential fatty acids. I recommend using olive and peanut oil for cooking. They are monounsaturates and can be heated to a rather high temperature before they break down and start smoking. Most of the recipes list them as the preferred oils to use.

Here are some low-fat cooking and eating tips:

- Use nonstick pans for cooking. They come in a variety of styles from skillets to baking sheets to muffin pans.
- Use the smallest possible amount of oil or margarine for sautéing. Sometimes ½ teaspoon will do when a recipe calls for ¼ cup. Wipe the oil across the pan with a paper towel or pastry brush. Even better, use a small amount of chicken or beef stock or the liquid from an ingredient you will add later, like canned tomatoes.
- Use a steamer rack for vegetables or cook them, partially covered, in a microwave for four to five

minutes with a spoon or two of water. It has the same effect as steaming. By the way, you lose the least amount of nutrients when cooking vegetables in a microwave. (However, you can't cook vegetables with tight skins like peas because they will burst as the steam builds up inside.)

- Trim all visible fat from meat before cooking. Broil or bake instead of frying. You can poach chicken or fish in broth or vegetable juice.
- Remove the skin from the chicken before you cook it unless you're roasting it (remove the skin from a roasted chicken after roasting). Sixty-two percent of the calories from chicken with the skin left on are from fat.
- Plan ahead when cooking soups or stews that contain fat. Allow them to cool (refrigerate if possible) and skim off the fat before you reheat and serve.
- Save all leftover chicken, turkey, and beef bones for broth. After simmering for several hours, refrigerate, and skim off the congealed fat. A quick method of cooling broth is to stir an ice cube or two into it. Another method for defatting broth is to pour it through a cheesecloth.
- When you buy meat, choose the leanest cuts. For beef, these include eye of round, round steak, chuck with round bone, flank steak, tenderloin, lean stew meat, and extra-lean ground beef. For pork, try pork loin or tenderloin, center-cut ham, and Canadian bacon. For lamb, use the leg, lamb steak, or sirloin chops. All cuts of veal are lean except the breast.

  Avoid processed meats like bologna, salami, sausage, and frankfurters. Leaner choices are sliced turkey breast, turkey ham, roast beef, any of the new, nearly fat-free versions of ham, chicken, and turkey cold cuts. Watch out for nitrates and nitrites that are used in processing since they have been reported to cause cancer. Check the label.
- Buy tuna packed in water, which saves you 200 fat calories per serving.
- Use low-fat milk at 120 calories per cup or, better yet,

skim milk at 80 calories per cup. Use evaporated skim milk for cooking.

- Despite its name, buttermilk is actually low in fat when made from low-fat or skim milk. Use it to replace milk in pancakes and baked goods (add ½ teaspoon of baking soda to the dry ingredients for each cup of buttermilk).
- In most recipes calling for sour cream, you can substitute plain nonfat yogurt and save 320 calories per cup. To keep yogurt from separating when cooking or stirring vigorously, first mix 1 tablespoon cornstarch and 1 tablespoon yogurt together, then stir into the yogurt you're using in the recipe. Always buy low-fat or, even better, nonfat yogurt.
- Use low-fat cottage cheese, ricotta, and part-skim mozzarella. Whipped cream cheese has one-third less fat then regular cream cheese, spreads more easily, and you may use less. Generally, use cheeses occasionally and sparingly.
- Use diet margarine. It contains half the fat of regular margarine. Whipped butter also contains less fat and fewer calories than regular butter.
- Try the new no-oil salad dressings or make your own.
- Buy "old-fashioned" or "natural" peanut butter that has no added sugar or hydrogenated oils.
- Eat more turkey. It's cheap and nutritious, and lower in fat than red meat.
- Eat more whole grains, cereals, beans, pasta, corn, starchy winter vegetables, and rice for complex carbohydrates, fiber, and protein minus fat and cholesterol.
- Try to include more fish in your diet. It's low in fat and calories and, as previously noted, the fish oils may help your heart. A study of 852 middle-aged men showed that eating fish once a day cut the death rate from heart attacks in half. Also, at Oregon Health Sciences University, 20 patients given a diet rich in fish oils had a 45-percent drop in cholesterol.

SUGAR AND SWEETENERS

Everyone knows diabetics shouldn't eat refined sugar. Foods like candy, jams and jellies, syrups, sugared gelatins, and cake frosting have to be avoided completely, unless they're being used to treat a reaction, of course. Your diabetic child can enjoy an occasional treat like ice cream or frozen yogurt when you use them as part of the allowed exchanges, but basically sugar intake should be kept to a minimum. Fortunately, there are artificial sweeteners to allow your child to enjoy a wider range of foods.

The difficult part of the sugar issue is often sibling and peer pressure. Depending on the age and attitude of your child, the problems can vary. Completely banning all sweets from the home may cause a family uprising, but there's a good middle ground you can walk and several paths to it.

When your child is first diagnosed, the family may, with firm resolve, decide to ban all sweets from the house. But as the novelty of diabetes wears off, the sweets may start reappearing. If your family has been used to iced cookies, overly sweet Danish and coffee cakes, and a freezer full of Sara Lee, you all have a tough job on your hands. But if your whole family wants to be in better health, in addition to supporting the diabetic member, some changes will need to be made. Here's some ammunition that may help.

Sugar provides *none* of the 44 nutrients essential to life. Currently, one-fifth to one-quarter of our daily calories comes from sugars that are added to foods. If you add the two-fifths of our daily calories that we eat as fats, that means we have to get 100 percent of our daily essential nutrients from just 40 percent of the calories we consume. Doesn't sound like a very smart diet, does it?

Americans are consuming more than 120 pounds of sugar a year per person. Sugar not only contains no nutrients; it also uses up vitamins and minerals in the process of being metabolized, adding up to a net loss of essential nutrients. To make matters worse, many heavily sweetened foods are also high in fat and are highly concentrated. A one-ounce candy bar contains the same amount of sugar (and three times the calories) as a five-ounce apple but takes up very little space in your stomach. It's easy to overeat when you have a well-developed sweet tooth.

The best thing you can do is wean your whole family from excess sugar. This can be accomplished by doing more home baking and purchasing fewer sweets. Keeping lots of fresh fruit in the house at all times helps. A box of beautiful ripe strawberries can be a special treat, as it is to my boys. You can also purchase foods that are treats but not sweetened. For example, bagels fresh from the bakery are a favorite at our house. Reducing sugar intake is a task to undertake gradually. Believe it or not, tastes do change. Some foods that were once gobbled up will now taste too sweet.

You can certainly allow siblings to have an occasional candy bar, but you might want to ask them to be sensitive to your diabetic child's feelings. Competition between siblings can be intense. For example, Brennan gets very upset when his brother, Robin, eats something Brennan can't, so Robin usually eats "forbidden" foods when Brennan's not around. Most parents I've interviewed have the whole family follow the same basic diet and do avoid eating forbidden foods in front of the diabetic family member. At the very least, they make sure they provide an acceptable alternative treat. I'm not advocating coddling a child with diabetes when it comes to "forbidden" foods. Our children must learn self-discipline, learn to say no, and learn to live in the real world, but family support and sensitivity are also vital.

Alternative foods bring us to the topic of artificial sweeteners. It's not easy having diabetes in our over-sweetened country. Thanks to the wonders of modern chemistry, we have ways to sweeten our foods other than by using sugar and its cousins, honey, molasses, corn syrup, etc. Whether these alternative sweeteners are good for us has been questioned. Saccharin has been shown to cause cancer in animals tested when fed in large amounts, but those studies haven't been directly correlated to humans yet. As a parent, it's hard to know what to do. We don't want to feed our children foods that might be carcinogenic. I think we need to look at those words *might be*. No one knows for certain that a child will get cancer from having a diet soda every day and a few saccharin-sweetened treats a week, but a child with diabetes who feels like an outcast because he can never eat the kinds of foods his friends eat is more likely to "cheat." As parents of diabetic children, we might not know for certain what saccharin will do; but we do know for certain what diabetes can do. We've heard the horror stories of blindness, kidney failure, and loss of limbs. It comes down to a trade-off, trading the uncertainties concerning artificial sweeteners for good blood sugar control and decreased possibilities of complications.

There are even some concerns about aspartame. It is suspected that ingesting a very large amount of it on a daily basis may create an imbalance. The imbalance may affect the neurological functions of the brain. The FDA has recommended that ingestion of aspartame be limited to 50 mg per kilogram of body weight. Loosely translated, that means one 12-ounce can of aspartame-sweetened soda per 12 pounds of body weight. For a four-year-old weighing 36 to 40 pounds, that means approximately three cans of soda a day. That may seem like a lot, but it might be easy to exceed the recommended limit when including items such as sugar-free gelatin and homemade Popsicles made from sugar-free drink mix.

Moderation is the key. Just as we don't want our other family members to have an overdeveloped sweet tooth, we don't want our diabetic child to have an overdeveloped artificial sweet tooth. In our house, I try to limit both the boys to one soda, diet or otherwise, a day. Desserts are rare treats. Usually once or twice a week we go out for frozen yogurt or ice cream. Many yogurt and ice cream parlors will supply calorie and carbohydrate information about their product. Use the method described in Chapter 2 under Label Reading to calculate exchanges. Using that information, I give Brennan a little extra insulin or have him eat less and use some of his meal or snack exchanges to cover the treat. You can discuss how to handle occasional departures from your child's diet with your dietitian.

Saccharin and aspartame are a little different in their chemical structure and their uses. Saccharin contains a molecule that the body views as a foreign substance and cannot be metabolized. It's sold under a variety of brand names such as SugarTwin and Sweet'n Low. It is used in baking but can leave a bitter aftertaste in large amounts.

Aspartame is marketed as NutraSweet and Equal. It is made up of two amino acids that are building blocks of protein. A scientist discovered it when he happened to lick his fingers while conducting an experiment and noticed a very sweet taste. A natural food element, it is metabolized normally by the body. It cannot be used for cooking since it breaks down at the boiling point (212°F) and loses its sweetness. Some people are sensitive to it and can experience dizziness and headaches. If that should happen, simply discontinue use. Call your doctor if you have any questions concerning this. Aspartame is not safe for the rare person who has PKU, an inability to process phenylalanine, one of the elements in aspartame.

Sorbitol and mannitol are sugar alcohols that metabolize in the same way as other sugars but are absorbed more slowly. They do, however, raise blood sugar and are not a basically "free" sweetener like saccharin or aspartame. Read the label of the food they sweeten and check calories and carbohydrate grams.

A quick word about fructose. Fructose is one of the sugars found in fruit. It can sometimes be used successfully as a sweetener for diabetics with excellent blood sugar control (most blood tests between 80 and 140). With adequate insulin in the body, the fructose will be stored as glycogen in the liver instead of entering the bloodstream as sugar. Several parents I interviewed use fructose for sweetening cookies and found it did not raise their children's blood sugars very much. Check with your dietitian.

SALT

Excluding sugar, salt is the nation's leading food additive. We consume over 15 pounds of salt a year per person in this country.

Salt is a potential killer for anyone who is sensitive to the blood-pressure-raising effects of sodium. Diabetic people need to be very cautious of anything that threatens their circulatory system since they already have an increased risk of heart disease due to diabetes. In addition, everyone in your family should be careful about sodium.

The biological need for salt is disputed, but may be as low as only about 220 milligrams of sodium daily, the equivalent of $\frac{1}{10}$ teaspoon of salt. The recommended intake is 1,100–3,300 milligrams of sodium for adults or the equivalent of $\frac{1}{2}$–$1\frac{1}{2}$ teaspoons of salt. Americans now consume between 2 and 4 teaspoons a day on the average.

The harmful effects of salt on blood pressure were first suggested in 1904. Studies among the Japanese, Eskimos, and Americans have shown a direct relationship between salt consumption and blood pressure. Even a study with six-month-old infants showed they had lower blood pressure when fed a low-sodium diet (breast milk only) than when fed a normal sodium diet of infant formulas and other foods.

Salt enters our diet in three ways. About one-third is naturally present in the foods we eat. Another third comes from salt we add to foods we are served. The final third comes from food processing. For example, one serving of an ordinary canned soup contains 1,000–1,500 milligrams of sodium. One fast-food meal of burger, fries, and a shake contains twice the recommended daily amount of sodium. An ounce of some breakfast cereals contains more sodium than the same amount of salted peanuts.

Human beings evolved on a diet that was not only low in sodium but also contained ample amounts of potassium. Potassium helps protect against high blood pressure and is found in fresh fruits and vegetables. The more processed foods (high in sodium) we eat, the less fresh food we eat. The message is clear. Eat foods as close to their natural state as possible. Fresh is best. The next choice should be frozen foods. Use canned goods infrequently. For example, I use only canned tomatoes and canned unsweetened pineapple in juice. Try the new low-sodium canned foods now available.

Get your family used to eating foods with less sodium. It's added insurance against heart disease. Here are some tips for lowering your salt intake:

1. If possible, rinse processed foods prepared with salt. Canned green beans and canned tuna are good examples.
2. Read labels. Sodium is also in brine, MSG, soy sauce, baking soda, and sodium citrate.
3. Reduce salty seasonings such as soy sauce, miso, barbecue sauce, garlic or onion salt, dry soup mixes, bouillon cubes, catsup, and oyster sauce. Use more herbs and spices, garlic and onion (fresh or powdered), fresh ginger, lemon, lime, vinegar, and wine. Worcestershire sauce has much less sodium than soy sauce. There is also a reduced-sodium soy sauce now marketed by Kikkoman. In regular soy sauce, Chun King's has 1,479 milligrams of sodium per tablespoon compared to 930 milligrams for Kikkoman's soy sauce.
4. Buy unsalted snacks. Crackers, potato chips, pretzels, and corn chips are now available without added

salt. Make your own popcorn and sprinkle on just a little salt or, better yet, none at all.

5. Try some of the new sodium-free seasoning or make your own with this American Heart Association mixture:

Herb Mix

½ teaspoon cayenne pepper
1 tablespoon garlic powder
1½ teaspoons each dried basil and parsley flakes
1¼ teaspoons each dried thyme and savory
1 teaspoon each onion powder, mace, and freshly ground black pepper

Put all ingredients in blender jar and blend until they are ground. Store indefinitely in an air-tight container.

Yield: ¼ cup

6. Remember that every ½ teaspoon of salt you add to a recipe adds 1,165 milligrams of sodium to the total. Divide that number by the number of servings and you'll know how much sodium you're adding in proportion.

7. Use homemade chicken and beef stock. Save bones in the freezer. When you have enough, put them in a soup pot and cover with water. Add a cut-up onion, a few sliced carrots, and a stalk or two of celery. Simmer for several hours. Strain, refrigerate, and then skim the fat. Store in your refrigerator or freezer and use as needed for soups, sauces, sautéing and cooking vegetables.

8. When using canned goods, look for "no added salt" or "reduced salt" foods. Introduce them gradually so your family has time to adjust. The taste for salt is a habit and can be retrained. I'm not suggesting you live salt-free, just that you will be much better off with a lower overall intake of sodium.

FIBER AND COMPLEX CARBOHYDRATES

Fiber is plant material that is resistant to digestion by human beings. It is found in unrefined grains (whole wheat, brown rice, etc.), dried beans, peas, fruits, and vegetables. In the last 30 years, the food industry has removed much of the plant fiber through processing, refining, and precooking. Nutritionists and health care professionals are now saying that fiber is important in the American diet and that we should eat more of it. There are many reasons for this.

On the whole, fibrous foods take longer to eat and, therefore, slow down the consumption of calories. Fiber is a filler-upper, taking space in your stomach and intestines. It absorbs water and slows down digestion so you feel full longer. In the large intestine, it helps eliminate solid wastes and more toxins out of the system more quickly. Most of the fiber is excreted, acting as a natural laxative. You are probably also aware that fiber is recommended to reduce the risk of colon cancer.

There are basically two types of fiber. One is the insoluble kind found in whole grains and bran. These fibers are identified as cellulose, hemicellulose, and lignins and are indigestible. Insoluble fiber adds bulk, holds water, and moves more food through the body. It assists in lowering overall blood cholesterol.

The other kinds of fiber are guar, pectins, and gums. They are water-soluble and are found in fruit, vegetables, beans, legumes, and cheap ice cream. They form a gel in the stomach and cause food to be held longer, resulting in a slower rise in blood sugar. Foods rich in starch and fiber such as oats, beans, and whole grain breads seem to increase the body's sensitivity to insulin and can sometimes lower insulin requirements. High-fiber food can also lower blood pressure and decrease blood-fat levels. This is important to people with diabetes as well as the general population.

Starchy foods high in fiber are also good sources of nutrients. The potato is a good example. A five-ounce potato provides only about 5 percent of the average adult's daily caloric needs but 6 percent of the protein; 8 percent folacin, phosphorus, and magnesium; 10 percent iron, niacin, and copper; 15 percent iodine; 20 percent vitamin B_6; 35 percent vitamin C; plus thiamine, riboflavin, and zinc. That's quite a nutritional bargain.

More and more athletes are turning away from the high-animal-protein diets to high-fiber and high-carbohydrate meals and finding improved performance. What's good for them is definitely good for all of us.

There are many easy ways to add complex carbohydrates and fiber to your diet:

1. Choose carbohydrates packaged in their natural coatings. Whenever possible, use brown rice instead of white, whole grain flour instead of white. Use whole grain crackers, breads, and cereals. Read labels. The term "wheat flour" is often used to describe bleached white flour. Look for the words whole wheat.

2. Choose fresh vegetables with edible skins and seeds such as tomatoes and cucumbers. Scrub but don't peel your carrots. Leave the skins on your potatoes. Steam vegetables with peels on.

3. Choose fruits with edible skins and seeds such as strawberries and apples. They can be raw or frozen or canned in juice, unsweetened. Eat whole fruit. Drink less juice.

4. Legumes can sometimes cause gas, so start with the most easily digested kind, such as lentils, split peas, and lima beans. Work up to including navy, pinto, kidney, and black beans.

5. Use whole grains such as barley, bulgur, and kasha as side dishes. Add wheat germ to meat loaf and meatballs. Make homemade corn bread and popcorn (air-popped or popped in the microwave without fat).

6. Oat bran is very helpful in lowering cholesterol and

blood-fat levels. It is available as a hot cereal and makes great muffins (see index).

7. Try to work up to 25–40 grams of fiber a day for each member of your family. Be aware that adding fiber may increase the need for fluids to avoid constipation problems. Check with your child's dietitian about the best way to incorporate fiber into his or her diet. Here are some examples:

FOOD	FIBER
fruits—1 FRUIT exchange	2 grams
vegetables—½–¾ cup cooked or 1–2 cups raw	2 grams
starchy vegetables—1 BREAD exchange	3 grams
legumes—1 BREAD exchange	8 grams
whole grain breads—1 BREAD exchange	2 grams
cereals—1 BREAD exchange	3 grams
bran cereals—1 BREAD exchange	8 grams
nuts and seeds—1 ounce—1 BREAD exchange	3 grams

8. Remember that soups are a great source of low-calorie, low-fat fiber and nutrition. There are many soup recipes in the lunch chapter in Part II. Don't be limited by the ingredients listed. Add extra vegetables you like. Use the exchange list in Chapter 2 to figure added food value.

9. Be aware that cooking vegetables until they're mush considerably lessens the fiber content.

Fiber may possibly interfere with the absorption of essential minerals. Minerals are excreted on a high-fiber diet, but how much is lost and the significance of that loss varies. Scientists at the United States Department of

Agriculture report that mineral losses from increased fiber are not significant for the average American consuming a well-balanced diet. Problems could potentially arise if a person's diet is already deficient in nutrients and is then further inhibited by excess fiber. This seems to indicate that for someone eating a well-balanced diet, adding fiber would be more beneficial than detrimental.

GLYCEMIC INDEX

You may have heard about glycemic index and be wondering what it means to your diabetic child. The truth is, we're not sure exactly what it means, and diets are not undergoing drastic changes because of it. However, it indicates we did not know as much as we thought we did about the way food affects blood sugar.

In the past, dietary recommendations were based on the chemical components of food. Now we have a method of judging how those foods are handled in the body. There is a wide variation, for example, in blood glucose response to BREAD exchange foods such as rice, legumes, corn, pasta, and wheat. The system of judging this response is called the *glycemic index*. It is devised by comparing each food to an equivalent amount of glucose. That results in a rating—100 being equal to a similar amount of glucose and on down the scale.

The idea is that a food with a 50 rating would raise blood sugar only half as much as one with a 100 rating. The problem is that the foods are being tested by themselves and sometimes in amounts that are far above serving portions. We don't know how this will change when they are part of a well-balanced meal. Some of the information is confusing, too. White potatoes raise blood sugar higher than ice cream, but you would be smarter to eat a potato every day than to eat ice cream from the standpoint of overall nutrition and health.

There are other factors to consider when discussing the glycemic index. The form of a food and the cooking process and time can also affect glycemic response. Studies have shown that the more a food is processed, the quicker the digestion of that food and the faster the rise in blood sugar. As examples, pureed vegetables raise blood sugar higher than chopped, chopped higher than whole, and cooked higher than raw.

In addition, the other foods eaten at a meal affect the body's response: the amount and type of fiber in the foods eaten, how much fat is in the food, the state of diabetes control, and the body's individual metabolism.

Based on the data available today, the best choices to make are low-fat, low-sugar, low-salt, high-fiber, and complex-carbohydrate foods. (Boy, that's a lot to remember.)

Simply put, choose foods as close to their natural state as possible while avoiding excess fats.

Nutritionists working in all fields are making the same basic recommendations. That's good news. It means you should feed your family the same basic diet you feed your diabetic child.

2
The Exchange Diet

Now that you've been inundated with the complexities of current nutrition trends, I turn your attention to the special needs of a person with diabetes and the exchange diet. (No one said this was going to be easy!)

I first became familiar with the idea of food exchanges after my second child, Robin, was born. I needed to lose 18 pounds and decided to try the Weight Watchers diet. I was nursing Robin at the time and took about four months to lose the weight. I noticed that the system of food exchanges or trades that Weight Watchers used was very easy. When Brennan was diagnosed two years later, the exchange diet seemed like an old friend.

In the exchange diet, food is divided into categories or classes, depending on the carbohydrate, protein, and fat content. Each type of food in the amounts listed has approximately the same composition and caloric content as the others in its class. It makes it easier to choose foods and make up balanced meals.

For example, starchy foods are generally listed under "BREAD Exchanges." They share the following characteristics.

Nutritive values per serving:	CAL	CHO (gm)	PRO (gm)	FAT (gm)
	70	15	2	0

These foods include breads, pasta, starchy vegetables, dried peas and beans, and cereals. At each meal, you

21

choose from any of the BREAD exchange items to fulfill
the allowed amount of exchanges in the diet plan.

All the food we eat can be classified as carbohydrate,
protein, fat, or a combination of these. Your child's insulin
dosage is probably based mostly on the amount of carbohydrate that has been allowed. That brings me to a very
important point.

There is no such thing as "better" or "worse" diabetes
when it comes to insulin dosage. There are three things
that do matter:

1. keeping good nutrition habits and eating balanced
   meals
2. maintaining ideal body weight
3. maintaining ideal blood sugar (80–150)

For example, your child has been taking two shots a day
of regular and NPH for a total of 25 units of insulin. After
a pattern of higher-than-normal tests develops, you and
your doctor decide to add a few units of regular or NPH to
the daily total. Don't feel that your child is now "sicker"
with diabetes because he's using more insulin. What
matters is balanced nutrition, body weight, and blood
sugars—the three Bs. It's the day-to-day consistency
that's important, and that's where the balance of insulin,
food, and exercise comes in.

The rest of the chapter is comprised of the six food
exchange categories and sample lists of common foods.
I've included exchanges for several popular fast-food restaurants. I also recommend the book *The Diabetic's
Brand Name Food Exchange Handbook*. It's written and
compiled by Andrea Barrett and published by Running
Press (Philadelphia, 1984). Your local American Diabetes
Association affiliate can supply you with additional exchange diet information.

The diet plan your child follows should be prepared by a
nutritionist, dietitian, diabetes nurse-educator, or other
diabetes specialist. If your doctor does not have someone
like this on his team, call the Juvenile Diabetes Founda-

tion or American Diabetes Association chapter nearest you and ask for a recommendation. Your child's diet plan will need to be updated as she grows. The more she weighs, the more calories she needs. In a growth spurt, for example, extra calories are imperative. Your child's hunger is the best gauge. Ideally, an annual diet plan update should be considered.

BREAD EXCHANGES

One BREAD exchange contains:	CAL	CHO (gm)	PRO (gm)	FAT (gm)
	70	15	2	0

The BREAD exchange list contains a wide variety of foods, including breads, cereals, starchy vegetables, and dried peas and beans. The quality of the nutrition and fiber you receive from this food group can vary a great deal. Those of us called health-food nuts 20 years ago for choosing whole grain breads and largely vegetable protein diets have recently been exonerated. Wise choices from this food category will make a difference in the overall health of your diabetic and your whole family. Once again, choose whole foods that have had a minimum of processing. Fifteen potato chips and one small baked potato are both counted as a BREAD exchange, but they share little else from the nutritional viewpoint. Look for whole wheat, whole grain bread products. Use soups made from dried peas and beans frequently. Serve a starchy vegetable with dinner instead of bread or rolls.

This list contains the foods and amounts that make up one BREAD exchange:

BREAD	AMOUNT
White (including French and Italian)	1 slice
Whole wheat	1 slice

Rye or pumpernickel	1 slice
Raisin	1 slice
Bagel	½
English muffin, small	½
Plain roll, bread	1
Frankfurter roll	½
Hamburger bun	½
Dried bread crumbs	3 tablespoons
Tortilla, 6 inches	1

CEREAL

These cereal products are all low-fat:

Bran flakes	½ cup
Buckwheat kasha (cooked)	½ cup
Bulgur (cooked)	¼ cup
Other ready-to-eat, unsweetened cereal	¾ cup
Puffed cereal (unfrosted)	1 cup
Cereal (cooked)	½ cup
Grits (cooked)	½ cup
Rice or barley (cooked)	½ cup
Pasta (cooked): spaghetti, noodles, macaroni	½ cup
Popcorn (popped, no fat added)	3 cups
Cornmeal (dry)	2 tablespoons
Flour	2½ tablespoons
Wheat germ	¼ cup

CRACKERS

Arrowroot	3
Graham (2½-inch square)	2
Matzo (4 inches by 6 inches)	½

Oyster	20
Pretzels (3⅛ inches long by ⅛ inch in diameter)	25
Rye wafers (2 inches by 3½ inches)	3
Saltines	6
Soda (2½-inch square)	4

DRIED BEANS, PEAS, AND LENTILS

Beans, peas, lentils (dried and cooked)	½ cup
Baked beans, no pork (canned)	¼ cup

STARCHY VEGETABLES

Corn	⅓ cup
Corn on the cob	1 small
Lima beans	½ cup
Parsnips	⅔ cup
Peas, green (canned or frozen)	½ cup
Potato, white	1 small
Potato (mashed)	½ cup
Pumpkin	¾ cup
Winter squash, acorn or butternut	½ cup
Yam or sweet potato	¼ cup

PREPARED FOODS

Biscuit (2-inch diameter) (add 1 FAT exchange)	1
Corn bread (2 inches by 2 inches by 1 inch) (add 1 FAT exchange)	1
Corn muffin (2-inch diameter) (add 1 FAT exchange)	1
Crackers, round butter-type (add 1 FAT exchange)	5

Pancake (5 inches by ½ inch)   1
   (add 1 FAT exchange)

Potatoes, French-fried (2–3½   8
   inches long) (add 1 FAT
   exchange)

Potato or corn chips (add 2   15
   FAT exchanges)

Waffle (5 inches by ½ inch)   1
   (add 1 FAT exchange)

FRUIT EXCHANGES

One FRUIT exchange contains:				
	CAL	CHO (gm)	PRO (gm)	FAT (gm)
	40	10	0	0

As much as possible, have your child eat whole fresh fruit. Use whatever is available at your market. Make a big fruit salad. It's a refreshing snack anytime. The next choice would be frozen fruit (without added sugar). Last choice from a nutrition standpoint is canned fruit. Fortunately, many fruits are now available water-packed and in unsweetened juices. Remember that the juice itself becomes a FRUIT exchange in serving portions of ⅓–½ cup.

This contains the commonly available foods and amounts that make up one FRUIT exchange:

FRUIT	AMOUNT
Apple	1 small
Apple juice	⅓ cup
Applesauce (unsweetened)	½ cup
Apricots, fresh	2 medium
Apricots, dried	4 halves
Banana	½ small
Blackberries	½ cup

Blueberries	½ cup
Cantaloupe	¼ small
Cherries	10 large
Cider	⅓ cup
Cranberries	Free
Dates	2
Figs, fresh	1
Figs, dried	1
Grapefruit	½
Grapefruit juice	½ cup
Grapes	12
Grape juice	¼ cup
Honeydew	⅛ medium
Lemon	1 large
Mango	½ small
Nectarine	1 small
Orange	1 small
Orange juice	½ cup
Papaya	¾ cup
Peach	1 medium
Pear	1 small
Persimmon	1 medium
Pineapple	½ cup
Pineapple juice	⅓ cup
Plums	2 medium
Prunes	2 medium
Prune juice	¼ cup
Raisins	2 tablespoons
Raspberries	½ cup
Strawberries	¾ cup
Tangerine	1 medium
Watermelon	1 cup

MILK EXCHANGES

One MILK exchange contains:	CAL	CHO (gm)	PRO (gm)	FAT (gm)
	80	12	8	trace

The best milk choices are those in the first list below, "Nonfat Fortified Milk." Because they are nonfat, these foods contain fewer calories.

NONFAT FORTIFIED MILK	AMOUNT
Skim or nonfat milk	1 cup
Powdered (nonfat dry, before adding liquid)	⅓ cup
Canned, evaporated skim milk	½ cup
Buttermilk made from skim milk	1 cup
Yogurt made from skim milk (plain, unflavored)	1 cup

LOW-FAT FORTIFIED MILK	
1%-fat fortified milk (add ½ FAT exchange and 22 calories)	1 cup
2%-fat fortified milk (add 1 FAT exchange and 45 calories)	1 cup
Yogurt made from 2%-fat fortified milk (plain, unflavored, add 1 FAT exchange and 45 calories)	1 cup

WHOLE MILK	
Whole milk (add 2 FAT exchanges and 90 calories)	1 cup
Canned evaporated whole milk (add 2 FAT exchanges and 90 calories)	½ cup

Buttermilk made from whole   1 cup
   milk (add 2 FAT exchanges
   and 90 calories)

Yogurt made from white milk   1 cup
   (plain, unflavored, add 2 FAT
   exchanges and 90 calories)

MEAT EXCHANGES

We've discussed the importance of plant fiber, but let me get in a word or two about excess animal protein. The American diet is considerably overburdened by animal protein. The average person eats twice as much protein as is needed for good nutrition.

I've included many recipes in this book that contain vegetables mixed in with animal protein sources. Try to serve red meat once or, at most, twice a week. Make all your protein sources low-fat choices and try for largely vegetable protein meals several times a week. Pasta dinners or a hearty soup with salad, vegetables, and homemade Irish soda bread are great possibilities (see index for recipes).

There are three types of MEAT exchanges: lean MEAT, medium-fat MEAT, and high-fat MEAT. Each is discussed below.

One lean MEAT exchange contains:	CAL	CHO (gm)	PRO (gm)	FAT (gm)
	55	0	7	3

The best choices for your family will be the proteins in this lean meat category. Be sure to trim any visible fat.

BEEF	
Baby beef (very lean)	1 ounce
Chipped beef	1 ounce
Chuck	1 ounce
Flank steak	1 ounce

LAMB

Leg	1 ounce
Rib	1 ounce
Sirloin	1 ounce
Loin (roast and chops)	1 ounce
Shank	1 ounce
Shoulder	1 ounce

PORK

Leg (whole rump, center, shank)	1 ounce
Ham	1 ounce
Smoked (center slices)	1 ounce

VEAL

Leg	1 ounce
Loin	1 ounce
Rib	1 ounce
Shank	1 ounce
Shoulder	1 ounce
Cutlets	1 ounce

POULTRY (all without skin)

Chicken	1 ounce
Cornish hen	1 ounce
Guinea hen	1 ounce
Pheasant	1 ounce
Turkey	1 ounce

FISH

Any fresh, frozen, or canned salmon, tuna, mackerel	1 ounce
Clams	5 or 1 ounce
Crab	¼ cup

Lobster	¼ cup
Oysters	5 or 1 ounce
Sardines (drained)	3
Scallops	5 or 1 ounce
Shrimp	5 or 1 ounce

CHEESE AND LEGUMES

Cheeses containing less than 5% butterfat	1 ounce
Cottage cheese, dry and 2% butterfat	1 ounce
Dried beans and peas (omit 1 BREAD exchange)	½ cup

One medium-fat MEAT exchange contains:	CAL	CHO (gm)	PRO (gm)	FAT (gm)
	75	0	7	5

BEEF

Ground (15% fat)	1 ounce
Corned beef (canned)	1 ounce
Rib eye	1 ounce
Round (ground commercial)	1 ounce

PORK

Boiled ham	1 ounce
Boston butt	1 ounce
Canadian bacon	1 ounce
Loin (all cuts tenderloin)	1 ounce
Shoulder arm (picnic)	1 ounce
Shoulder blade	1 ounce

HIGH-CHOLESTEROL MEAT EXCHANGES

Cottage cheese, creamed	¼ cup
Egg (high in cholesterol)	1

Heart	1 ounce
Kidney	1 ounce
Liver	1 ounce
Sweetbreads	1 ounce

CHEESE

Farmer's	1 ounce
Mozzarella	1 ounce
Neufchâtel	1 ounce
Parmesan	3 tablespoons
Ricotta	1 ounce

MISC.

Peanut butter (omit 2 FAT exchanges)	2 tablespoons

One high-fat MEAT exchange contains:	CAL	CHO (gm)	PRO (gm)	FAT (gm)
	100	0	7	8

BEEF

Beef brisket	1 ounce
Chuck (ground commercial)	1 ounce
Corned beef (brisket)	1 ounce
Ground beef (more than 20% fat)	1 ounce
Roasts (rib)	1 ounce
Steaks (club and rib)	1 ounce

LAMB

Breast	1 ounce

PORK

Country-style ham	1 ounce
Deviled ham	1 ounce

Ground	1 ounce
Loin (back ribs)	1 ounce
Spareribs	1 ounce

VEAL

Breast	1 ounce

POULTRY

Capon	1 ounce
Duck (domestic)	1 ounce
Goose	1 ounce

CHEESE

Cheddar types	1 ounce

PROCESSED MEATS

Cold cuts (4¼ inches by ⅛ inch)	1 slice
Frankfurter (1 of 10 in a 16-ounce package)	1 small

VEGETABLE EXCHANGES

One VEGETABLE exchange contains:	CAL	CHO (gm)	PRO (gm)	FAT (gm)
	25	5	2	0

Vegetables in this list are among the best health bargains you can get your child to eat. Don't skimp on them. Your dietitian may put down two VEGETABLE exchanges for your child's dinner, but if your child wants more, it's a good idea to provide them for several reasons.

First of all, they fill your child with fiber. Remember the nutrition information about fiber? It slows down the rise of blood sugar because food takes longer to digest. Of course, the vegetables need to be raw or lightly steamed for the fiber to have its fullest effect. Tomato sauce has almost no fiber at all and can cause blood sugar to rise. As a matter of fact, $\frac{2}{3}$ cup of tomato sauce counts as a BREAD. The same would apply to mashed or pureed vegetables. But raw or lightly cooked vegetables could be said to have almost a negative effect on blood sugar. Remember to include any fats from salad dressings or cooking that cling to these healthy goodies. One exchange is $\frac{1}{2}$ cup, cooked or raw.

Asparagus
Bean sprouts
Beets
Broccoli
Brussels sprouts
Cabbage, red/green
Carrots
Cauliflower
Celery
Chinese pea pods
Eggplant
Green onions
Green pepper
Greens:
    Beet
    Chards
    Collards
    Dandelion
    Kale
    Mustard
    Spinach
    Turnip
Mushrooms
Okra
Onion
Rhubarb
Rutabaga
Sauerkraut
String beans, green/yellow

Summer squash
Tomatoes
Tomato catsup (2 tablespoons)
Tomato juice
Turnips
Vegetable juice
Zucchini

The following raw vegetables may be used as desired (free):

Chicory
Chinese cabbage
Cucumber
Endive
Escarole
Lettuce
Parsley
Pepper, green/red
Pickles, dill
Radishes
Watercress

FAT EXCHANGES

One FAT exchange contains:	CAL	CHO (gm)	PRO (gm)	FAT (gm)
	45	0	0	5

The following foods count as one FAT exchange. The capitalized choices are low in saturated fats.

MISC.	AMOUNT
MARGARINE, SOFT, TUB, OR STICK*	1 teaspoon
AVOCADO (4-inch diameter)	⅛

OILS

CORN	1 teaspoon
COTTONSEED	1 teaspoon
OLIVE**	1 teaspoon
PEANUT**	1 teaspoon
SAFFLOWER	1 teaspoon
SOYBEAN	1 teaspoon
SUNFLOWER	1 teaspoon

NUTS

OLIVES**	5 small
ALMONDS**	10 whole
PECANS**	2 whole large
PEANUTS**	
SPANISH	20 whole
VIRGINIA	10 whole
WALNUTS	6 small
OTHER NUTS	6 small

*Made with corn, cottonseed, safflower, soy, or sunflower oil only.
**Fat content is primarily monounsaturated.

Bacon, crisp	1 strip
Bacon fat	1 teaspoon
Butter	1 teapsoon
Cream	
Heavy	1 tablespoon
Light	2 tablespoons
Sour	2 tablespoons
French dressing†	1 tablespoon
Italian dressing†	1 tablespoon
Lard	1 teaspoon
Margarine, stick	1 teaspoon
Mayonnaise†	1 teaspoon

| Salad dressing (mayonnaise type)† | 2 teaspoons |
| Salt pork | ¾-inch cube |

---

†Preferably made with corn, cottonseed, safflower, soy, or sunflower oil.

FAST FOODS

If you have a child, you can't escape fast-food restaurants. Fast foods are far from nutritionally ideal, but eating them occasionally is not going to harm your child.

Be aware that most of the foods offered are high in fat, sodium, and calories. For example, Burger King's chicken sandwich has 42 grams of fat, 775 milligrams of sodium, and 690 calories! It counts as 3½ BREAD, 3 lean MEAT, and 6½ FAT. Kentucky Fried Chicken's mashed potatoes, gravy, coleslaw, and roll adds up to 3 BREAD, 3½ medium-fat MEAT, and 3 FAT, with 1,528 milligrams of sodium and 604 calories. These foods are woefully short on fiber, too.

Fortunately, many fast-food establishments now offer baked potatoes and salad bars. Just be sure to watch the toppings and salad dressings, which add fat and calories.

Try to get your child to stick to simpler fare—a hamburger instead of a Whopper or Big Mac, a small order of fries, and a diet soda. A meal like that would be approximately 3½–4 BREAD, 2 medium-fat MEAT, and 2–3 FAT.

For an extensive listing of fast-food nutrients and exchanges, send for *FAST FOOD FACTS*, © 1985 by the International Diabetes Center, 5000 West 39th Street, Minneapolis, MN 55416. The booklet is available for $2.50 plus $.75 for postage and handling.

LABEL READING

Thanks to consumer groups and the current interest in nutrition, quite a lot of basic nutrition information is now listed on food packages. Labels don't list food exchanges, but you can determine that yourself with just a little practice. Just read the label and use the following techniques. Ask these questions:

1. Of what foods is the purchased item comprised? What are the ingredients, or what does it most resemble?
2. Check the nutritional information and see if the item contains mostly carbohydrate, protein, or fats.
3. See if the ingredients' exchanges add up to the listed protein, carbohydrate, and fat grams on the label.

I know that sounds confusing, but I'll show you how it works. I took three items out of my refrigerator that have nutrition information. They were Weight Watchers' Spaghetti with Meat Sauce, Weight Watchers' Pepperoni Pizza (individual serving size), and Alta-Dena Nonfat Black Cherry Yogurt. Let's figure the exchanges.

WEIGHT WATCHERS' SPAGHETTI WITH MEAT SAUCE

1. What does it most resemble? What are the ingredients? Well, it's basically pasta, which counts as a BREAD, and meat sauce, which counts as a MEAT, plus tomatoes, a VEGETABLE.
2. What is the main nutritional element? This food has 36 grams carbohydrates, 16 grams protein, and 8 grams fat. Answer: CARBOHYDRATES.

Since spaghetti is the main ingredient, and spaghetti is a BREAD exchange, let's see how BREAD fits into the nutritional information we have. We're guessing to see if one or two BREAD exchanges fit this dish.

	1 BREAD	2 BREAD	SPAGHETTI WITH MEAT SAUCE
CHO:	15	30	36

| PRO: | 2 | 4 | 16 |
| FAT: | 0 | 0 | 8 |

Now deduct 2 BREAD from the listed grams.

	SPAGHETTI		2 BREAD		
CHO:	36	–	30	=	6 grams
PRO:	16	–	4	=	12 grams
FAT:	8	–	0	=	8 grams

What other food is in this dish? Meat. OK, 1 medium-fat MEAT exchange is:

CHO: 0 grams
PRO: 7 grams
FAT: 5 grams

Compare 2 medium-fat MEAT exchanges to the leftover grams above:

2 MEDIUM-FAT MEAT EXCHANGES	SPAGHETTI
CHO: 0 grams	6 grams
PRO: 14 grams	12 grams
FAT: 10 grams	8 grams

Now you know the spaghetti dish has 2 BREAD exchanges and almost 2 medium-fat MEAT exchanges. What about the extra carbohydrates? Well, the other main ingredient is tomato sauce, and tomatoes are counted as a VEGETABLE. One VEGETABLE exchange is:

CHO: 5 grams
PRO: 2 grams
FAT: 0 grams

The 5 grams of carbohydrate nearly match the 6 grams left after the BREADS and MEATS were deducted. So Weight Watchers' Spaghetti with Meat Sauce is approximately 2 BREAD, 2 medium-fat MEAT, and 1 VEGETABLE. Don't you feel smart? I do. I never knew how to do this until I wrote this book!

Let's try another.

WEIGHT WATCHERS' PEPPERONI PIZZA

370 calories
1 serving per container (That means the information is based on
the whole package. Always check the serving size.)
CHO: 38 grams
PRO: 21 grams
FAT: 15 grams

Pizza is comprised of bread dough and tomato sauce.
This one also has pepperoni, a very fatty meat. Now, 2
BREAD exchanges would be a good place to start since
the pizza is mostly bread dough.

	PIZZA		2 BREAD		
CHO:	38	—	30	=	8 grams
PRO:	21	—	4	=	17 grams
FAT:	15	—	0	=	15 grams

Now we see that we have protein and fat that need to fit
into some exchanges. Aha, the pepperoni! So we look at
high-fat MEAT:

	PIZZA LEFTOVERS		2 HIGH-FAT MEAT		
CHO:	8	—	0	=	8 grams
PRO:	17	—	14	=	3 grams
FAT:	15	—	16	=	−1 gram

We've used 2 BREAD, and 2 high-fat MEAT exchanges.
The leftover 8 grams of carbohydrates and 3 grams of
protein approximately fit one VEGETABLE exchange of 5
grams of carbohydrates and 2 grams of protein. TOTAL: 2
BREAD, 2 high-fat MEAT, 1 VEGETABLE.

A quick note: Because the tomato sauce is highly concentrated with no fiber in it, it could also be counted as a
BREAD. Check with your dietitian.

One last quick one:

ALTA-DENA NONFAT BLACK CHERRY YOGURT

Ingredients: Basically milk and fruit.
Serving size: 1 cup
1 serving per container
190 calories
CHO: 35 grams
PRO: 13 grams
FAT: less than 1 gram

1 MILK and 2 FRUIT would be:

CHO:	12	+	20	=	32
PRO:	8	+	0	=	8
FAT:	trace	+	0	=	trace

Subtract them from the yogurt.

	YOGURT		MILK/FRUIT		
CHO:	35	−	32	=	3 grams
PRO:	13	−	8	=	5 grams
FAT:	trace	−	trace	=	0 grams

The leftovers don't fit any easy pattern. They most closely resemble ½ MILK at 6 grams carbohydrate and 4 grams protein. So the total would be approximately 2 FRUIT and 1½ MILK exchanges.

In your kitchen, keep a one-page chart listing the carbohydrate, protein, and fat breakdown of each exchange as a quick reference. Good luck!

3
Stocking Your Kitchen

There are two elements you need to prepare nutritious meals for your family—the right ingredients and the appropriate equipment. This chapter is simply a list of suggested foods and utensils that you can use to compare to your present kitchen stockpile.

FOODS FOR A HEALTHY KITCHEN

The foods listed below are ones that I always keep on hand. They give me the freedom to cook the many recipes in this book. Many of these ingredients appear again and again. If you've never used a particular item, buy a small quantity and give it a try. Change comes slowly!

FLOURS AND GRAINS

Unbleached all-purpose white flour
Stone-ground whole wheat flour
Stone-ground cornmeal
Wheat germ (toasted or raw)
Whole wheat pastry flour
Old-fashioned rolled oats (for cereal and baking)
Bread crumbs (you can make your own and store in the refrigerator)
Barley (for soups and as a side dish)
Brown long-grain rice

43

Chinese or Korean rice (not instant)
Popcorn

LEAVENING AND THICKENERS

Baking powder, double-acting
Baking soda
Active dry yeast
Cornstarch
Unflavored gelatin
Arrowroot

DRY SEASONINGS

Allspice
Aniseed
Basil leaves
Bay leaves
Cayenne pepper
Celery seed
Chili powder
Cinnamon, sticks and ground
Cloves, whole and ground
Cocoa powder, unsweetened
Coriander
Cumin
Curry powder
Dill weed
Fennel seed
Garlic powder
Ginger, ground
Mace
Marjoram
Mint leaves
Mustard, dry
Nutmeg, ground (try buying the whole
    nutmeg and grating it as needed)
Oregano leaves

Paprika
Parsley flakes (use only if you can't get it
    fresh)
Black peppercorns
Rosemary
Sage
Salt
Sesame seeds, hulled
Sugars
Sweeteners, saccharin-type for baking
    (Sweet'n Low, SugarTwin, and Brown
    SugarTwin) and Equal (I use packets—
    approximately one gram—and bulk
    packages)
Tarragon
Cream of tartar (for beating egg whites)
Thyme leaves
Turmeric
White peppercorns (a delicate flavor on
    vegetables and in sauces)

WET SEASONINGS

Almond extract
Capers (they're salty)
Catsup
Garlic, one or more heads (store in dry, cool
    place)
Gingerroot, fresh, small piece
Honey (for baking)
Horseradish (prepared without additives)
Mayonnaise, diet and regular
Molasses, blackstrap (for baking)
Mustard, yellow or brown
Sherry, dry and cream (for cooking)
Soy sauce, low-sodium preferred
Vanilla extract
Vinegars, white, cider, white wine, red wine,
    and rice

White wine, dry (for cooking)
Worcestershire sauce

OILS

Corn, sunflower, or safflower (for cooking
    and salads)
Olive oil (Try extra virgin. It's mild and from
    the first pressing.)
Peanut oil (refrigerate)
Sesame oil (dark Oriental type)

BASIC INGREDIENTS TO HAVE ON HAND

Beans and peas, dried: pinto, red, lentils, split
    peas, etc.
Buttermilk, liquid or powdered (for baking)
Bread, whole-grain
Carrots
Celery
Cheeses for grating: Cheddar, Swiss,
    Parmesan, Gruyère
Cottage cheese, low-fat
Evaporated skim milk
Flavored diet-drink mixes (like Crystal Light)
Jam, low-sugar
Lemons
Margarine, diet
Milk, low-fat or skim and nonfat dry instant
Mineral waters and seltzer
Nuts: walnuts, pecans, almonds
Onions, yellow all-purpose
Oranges and orange juice (frozen
    unsweetened)
Pasta, lots of varieties
Peanut butter, natural, no sugar or
    hydrogenated oils
Potatoes, all-purpose (russets)

Raisins, seedless black and golden
Soft drinks, diet and flavored
Sugarless cocoa mix, commercial or
  homemade
Sugarless flavored gelatin
Sugarless pudding mix
Tea, herbal (orange spice, chamomile, mint)
Tomato paste and sauce, a few cans of each
Tomatoes, canned and peeled, in juice or
  puree, various size cans
Yogurt, nonfat plain or low-fat

KITCHEN EQUIPMENT

The following equipment will help you fulfill your potential as a chef and chief nutritionist. It is meant to give you ideas for equipment you might consider useful. If your family is going through changes in diet as a group, it's best to get them all involved. The children can help with a shopping expedition for new utensils and food items. Both parents and children can work together to achieve a new, satisfying level of culinary excellence.

KNIVES

Good, sharp ones—carbon steel are a good investment. They keep an edge better than most.

Paring knife: a 2- to 4-inch blade for delicate
  cutting
Chef's knife: heavy, for most cutting,
  chopping, and slicing
Bread knife: long, serrated blade for slicing
  bread and tomatoes
Utility knife: a 6- to 8-inch blade for boning
  chicken, cutting small vegetables
Grapefruit knife: The curved blade comes in
  handy for a number of uses.

POTS AND PANS AND BAKING DISHES

Assorted sizes with lids, preferably nonstick. Silverstone is better than Teflon.

> Stockpot: 8 quarts for pasta and soups. I have a handy one that has two steamers that fit inside it. It's called a *pasta pot*. I use it at almost every meal.
>
> Wok: You can use a skillet, but a wok is really great to have. A 12-inch-diameter size is a good size. I find I cook more meals and vegetables the healthy, Oriental way since buying it.
>
> Roasting pan with a cover
>
> Kettle for boiling water
>
> Steamer rack (or get the pasta/steamer pot mentioned above)
>
> Nonstick cookie sheets
>
> Baking pans: Ovenproof glass or ceramic is a good choice; 8- by 8- by 2-inch and 13- by 9- by 2-inch sizes
>
> Loaf pans: at least 2; glass bakes faster
>
> Muffin tins: with 12 cups, preferably nonstick
>
> Pie plates: it's good to keep 2 on hand.
>
> Baker's rack for cooling bread and cookies
>
> Casseroles with covers: 1½- and 3-quart sizes

UTENSILS AND SUCH

Eggbeater or small electric mixer

Spatulas

Wooden spoons: 2 or 3 different sizes

Slotted spoon

Ladle for soups

Juicer: hand variety or electric

Funnel with screw-on adapters for wide and narrow necks and a strainer

Rolling pin

Measuring cups and spoons

Mixing bowls: Pyrex or ceramic or stainless
  steel

Grater: one four-sided with various grates
  and one very fine one for nutmeg

Fine-mesh strainers

Large colander

Can opener: I like the manual Swing-Away
  one. I've found it very reliable.

Bottle and juice can opener

Corkscrew

Tongs for odd-shaped food items

Long-handled fork

Pepper mill for the freshest ground pepper

Pastry brushes for pastry and for oiling pans

Cutting board

Kitchen scissors for snipping herbs

Cheesecloth for fine straining

Mortar with pestle for grinding spices and
  herbs: preferably ceramic

Garlic press

Cheese slicer: It cuts very thin slices and
  helps cut down on saturated fats.

Fat-separating cup: The spout originates at
  the bottom so the liquid is poured off while
  the fat remains. A very handy item for a
  low-fat kitchen.

Grapefruit spoons: less work if you have
  grapefruit eaters

Pasta rake: a spoonlike paddle with forklike
  projections that's good for stirring and
  serving pasta

Marble slab: This is a luxury for the chef who
  kneads bread and rolls pastry, much better
  than wood.

Ice cream scoops: Use them for rice and
  grains as well as homemade low-calorie

sherberts.

Mallet for flattening and tenderizing chicken and meat

APPLIANCES

Blender and/or food processor: At least have a blender if you can. The food processor is handy; I use it all the time too.

Microwave: It's not essential but really handy. I find it great for reheating, defrosting, and cooking vegetables.

Toaster oven: It's an energy saver for baking a few potatoes or small portions as well as toasting.

Hot-air corn popper (or use the microwave)

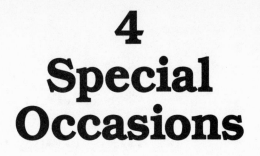

4
Special
Occasions

An important part of good diabetes management is day-to-day consistency. Holidays and parties can feel like a threat to good control. They don't have to be. Knowing how to combine insulin, food, exercise, and understanding can help you be flexible enough for any special occasion. Diversionary tactics help, too!

The information in this chapter is based on advice from professionals and the experiences of other parents, including me.

CAMPING

A family camping trip is a great source of exercise and relaxation. It just takes a little extra planning when you have a diabetic along.

Remember that with increased exercise comes increased need for calories. The caloric output can increase from 2,000 to 3,000 calories a day because of hiking, bicycling, etc. Discuss adjusting your child's food intake and insulin dosage with your health professional. Be sure to have plenty of food handy. The following foods are examples of meal and snack possibilities.

BREAKFAST

Canned fruit juices	½ cup = 1 FRUIT
Dried fruit	¼ cup = 1 FRUIT
Eggs	dried, 2 tablespoons = 1 medium-fat MEAT

51

Canned meats	1 ounce = 1 high-fat MEAT
Granola	¼ cup = 1 BREAD
Cooked cereal	½ cup = 1 BREAD
Biscuits	2-inch = 1 BREAD, 1 FAT
Corn bread	2-inch squares = 1 BREAD, 1 FAT
Pancakes	3–4-inch = 2 BREAD, 1 FAT
French toast	1 slice = 1 BREAD, ½ MEAT
Cocoa (sugarless)	1 cup = 1 MILK

LUNCH OR SNACKS

Raisins	2 tablespoons = 1 FRUIT
RY KRISP	3 triple crackers = 1 BREAD
Soda crackers	4–5 = 1 BREAD, 1 FAT
Popcorn	3 cups = 1 BREAD
Sunflower or pumpkin seeds	1 teaspoon = 1 medium-fat MEAT
Peanut butter	2 tablespoons = 1 medium-fat MEAT, 2 FAT
Trail mix (without chocolate)	⅓ cup = 1 BREAD, 1 FAT
Graham crackers	2 squares = 1 BREAD
Hard salami	¼-inch slice = 1 high-fat MEAT
Cheese	1 ounce = 1 high-fat MEAT

DINNER

| Casserole of macaroni and cheese, tuna and noodles, spaghetti and meat sauce | 1 cup = 2 BREAD, 2 MEAT, 1–2 FAT |
| Vegetables, dried | 1 ounce dried = 1 VEGETABLE |

You'll probably choose a campsite where some medical help is locally available, but be completely prepared anyway. Take two bottles of each insulin your child uses with lots of syringes. Be sure to take glucagon and the appropriate syringe. (Remember, it does have to be kept refrigerated.) Rehearse the steps of loading and mixing glucagon so they are current in your mind. Take goodies for insulin reactions like cake-gel (frosting in a tube) or

Glutose. Cans of juice, little boxes of raisins, and packages of cheese and crackers are also good to have along. Blood-testing becomes even more important as schedules change, so take along everything you need and more. Divide the supplies into a few different locations. Make sure they are well padded and out of direct sunlight. Everything will probably go very smoothly, but you'll feel much better knowing you have everything you need.

Talk with your doctor and/or diabetes educator to see if there's anything special you should know. Make sure your child has a medical identification bracelet or pendant in case you should be separated. They are available from Medic Alert Foundation International in Turlock, California 95381-1009, for a $20 lifetime membership.

HOLIDAYS

Holidays mean food, and that means careful planning and some adjusting for your child and, hopefully, your family. I've included several recipes in the dinner chapter in Part II that can be used for holiday meals. See the index to locate the following potential holiday recipes. Use the master list of recipes before the index to find more possibilities.

Roast Turkey with Stuffing
Noodle Kugel
Stuffed Yams
Puffed Sweet Potatoes
Mashed Turnips
Hash Brown Turnips
Carrot-Acorn Squash
Squash with Apples
Fruit Spiced Carrots
Corn Pudding
Cherry Pie
All-American Cranberry Sauce
Cranberry Relish
Cranberry Mold

Cran-Apple Crisp
Easy Sugarless Pumpkin Pie

A sample holiday menu might be:

Roast Turkey with Stuffing	5 lean MEAT, 1⅔ BREAD
Mashed Turnips	1½ VEGETABLE
Fruit Spiced Carrots	2 VEGETABLE
Cranberry Relish	½ FRUIT (up to 4 tablespoons free)
Pumpkin Pie	½ MILK, 1½ BREAD, 1 FAT

For Halloween, you needn't ban your child from trick-or-treating. You just need to make an agreement beforehand that nothing will be eaten until the bag comes home. Then separate the candy from the "OK" goodies—apples, raisins, sugarless gum, pennies. Trade the candy for cash and a trip to the toy store. Or try replacing it with sugarless candy. Have your child collect for the Juvenile Diabetes Foundation. It has a campaign called "Treat a kid who can't have a treat." The money goes to research to find a cure. You could also discuss sharing the candy with others. For example, I take all the Halloween treats into the studio and let *them* worry about their waistlines. Most of all, get it out of the house.

For Christmas and Thanksgiving, you can discuss with your dietitian or doctor whether to increase insulin or stick to the regular diet plan. If there are a lot of sweets around the house, have some alternative choices that are appropriate. The Pumpkin Pie and Cranberry Mold recipes (see index) are ones that everyone can enjoy. Try to make the holiday time a "people" time, not a time that's defined by foods only.

For Easter baskets, use colored eggs, sugarless gum, sugarless candies, and little toys or favors.

PARTIES

Whether the party is at your house or someone else's, it requires extra thought and planning.

If the party is in your home, you can control what foods are served. You don't have to serve candy for a party to be a success. I serve chips and dip, carrot sticks, little boxes of raisins, and an ice cream cake. I use sugarless drink mixes like Crystal Light. The kids don't care as long as it tastes good to them. We make exercise and games part of any party. One year we had everyone bring tennis shoes and we had a big free-for-all soccer game on the tennis court. The winning team got prizes. Then we had a Junior Trivia contest. The winner got a toy. Another year we played Bingo. They had a great time.

If you're serving lunch, you can make stacks of peanut butter and low-sugar jam sandwiches, baked chicken legs (the oven-fried kind), and tuna and egg salad sandwiches.

I also put out a bowl of fruit like plums or seedless green grapes, and they are always gobbled up.

If you don't feel like cooking, you can order from the local fast-food establishment and supplement with fresh fruit and cut-up veggies and dip. Believe it or not, kids will eat foods that are good for them even at a birthday party.

If the party is not in your home, the manner in which you handle it will depend on the age of your child. An adolescent will not want mom or dad interfering in his social life, but with a younger child, you will want to call the hosts and see what foods are being served. You can then discuss the choices beforehand with your child. A small piece of cake without icing would probably count as 1½ to 2 BREAD and 1 FAT. One small scoop of ice cream would be approximately 1 BREAD, 2 FAT. You might need to check with your dietitian or doctor to see about increasing the insulin so that your child can enjoy some of the allowable treats. In your conversation with the hosts, you might offer to bring any special foods or drinks your child would need. For example, you could bring diet sodas or sugarless drink mix if they'd planned on having only sugared drinks.

A party is a good learning opportunity for your child. He can learn how to make appropriate choices and be responsible for his diabetes while seeing that diabetes control can be flexible enough to allow him to be a kid and have fun.

I got a letter from a nine-year-old girl recently who wanted a recipe for a sugarless cake everyone would like that she could serve at her birthday party. Her best friend had diabetes and the friend's mother never let her go to parties where "bad" foods were served. My heart ached for her little friend. Her friend could easily have worked a small piece of cake (with icing removed) and/or a scoop of ice cream into her diet plan or covered it with a little extra insulin. The mother could have tested her daughter's blood sugar an hour or two after the party. If it were higher than acceptable, she could have consulted her doctor and used a combination of exercise and/or insulin to bring it down.

I remember one time, Brennan ate the fudge icing (while I wasn't looking!) off the ice cream cake at his birthday party and didn't tell me. About two hours later, after the party ended, I tested him. He had an 820 blood sugar! He and I looked at each other, and our eyes filled up with tears. He was scared. He told me he had eaten the icing. I called his doctor, got advice on increased dosage, and gave him his shot. I then sent him out to play basketball for an hour. After that hour, his blood sugar had dropped to 220. I waited thirty minutes more and gave him a light dinner. That was the last time he ate icing! That also gives you an example of how effective insulin and exercise can be in bringing down a high blood sugar.

No matter what your child's age, be sure he knows which foods he can eat and which he should not. Provide lots of positive reinforcement for his making the appropriate choices.

RESTAURANTS

Eating out with a diabetic child doesn't have to be a problem. It just takes some planning and some common sense. Here are some tips that will help.

1. In Part III, "The Copebook," I discuss the importance of waiting at least 15 to 20 minutes between the insulin injection and eating. When dining out, you might try checking the blood sugar at home just before leaving for the restaurant. Then you could give the insulin at the restaurant just before or after you order. If your child starts to feel low, she could have some juice and a few crackers until dinner arrives. If the dinner is unreasonably delayed, don't be shy about telling the waiter or hostess that you need to have the food served right away.

2. If the portions are too large, ask for a doggie bag and take some home.

3. Carry pocket- or purse-sized cards of the food exchange lists for a handy reference if you need them.

4. Watch for hidden fats. Fried foods, cream sauces, salad dressings, gravies, lots of mayonnaise on a sandwich are all bad for diabetic diets and everyone's health. Assist your child in choosing low-fat foods. Ask how a dish is prepared if you're not sure. Many restaurants offer foods that are lower in fat and follow the recommendations of the American Heart Association.

5. Fresh fruit or a small serving of sherbert or ice cream is a good choice for dessert.

6. Check to see if the restaurant carries diet drinks if you let your child have them with meals. If not, bring your own. Also, many restaurants carry low-fat or skim milk.

7. Take eating out as an opportunity for your child to make choices based on his diet plan. If he's allowed 2 BREAD exchanges, he should be aware that two rolls eaten before dinner is served will mean he can't eat the potatoes or rice served. Giving your child control of these diet decisions as early in life as possible helps the child to feel some sense of control over his diabetes.

SPORTS

There are two ways to attend a sporting event, as a participant and as a spectator. Each requires some planning.

If your child is a participant, there are several factors of which to be aware. One is the time of the event and which insulin will be working. If it's at 10:00 A.M., your child's regular insulin will be peaking. You can give a little less insulin and a little extra food. For example, when Brennan has a morning game, I give him less regular insulin, make sure he has a hearty breakfast, and see that he has orange juice available all during the game. If he has an afternoon game, I give less NPH and more food. There's another factor to consider. Adrenaline can cause a rise in blood sugar. Your child's getting excited at a game could cause him to have higher blood sugar even though he's exercising. Each child responds differently to excitement and anxiety. Discuss your child's individual reactions with your educator or doctor. Keeping close track of blood sugars will give you the information you need to decide what to do.

Whether or not you change the insulin dose, be sure to have your blood-testing equipment close. It's always a good idea to test blood sugar before exercising and provide extra food as needed. Also have a supply of foods to treat reactions, like fruit juices, Dextrasol tabs, or cake-gel for immediate sugar and cheese and crackers to follow up a reaction with protein and carbohydrates. You can provide a bottle with half water and half juice that your child can sip during the game. Your dietitian can provide additional ideas. By the way, your child should be taught to carry some source of glucose with him at all times. Be sure coaches and gym teachers are aware of the symptoms of insulin reactions and know how to treat them.

Being a spectator merely means dealing with all the less-than-healthy food at the baseball or football game.

Here are some foods you'd commonly buy at sporting events. They're almost all high in fat. If your child will be there at mealtime, you might take along a few healthy foods like carrot sticks and fresh fruit.

Beef frankfurter with bun	1½ BREAD, ½ MEAT, 2½ FAT
Hamburger (¼ pound) with bun	2 BREAD, 2 MEAT, 1½ FAT
Small order fries	2 BREAD, 2 FAT
Popcorn (approx. 2 cups)	1 BREAD, 1½ FAT
Peanuts, roasted in the shell (1 ounce)	½ MEAT, 2 FAT

PART II
THE COOKBOOK

5
Introduction to Recipes

The recipes in this section are designed to suit the diets of diabetic children, but they're also intended to appeal to your whole family's taste buds. Every parent and health professional I interviewed felt the whole family should eat the same basic meals as the diabetic child. The psychological support of eating the same foods greatly reduced the stress of "being different." Of course, an even better reason is that it's a very healthy way to eat. These recipes make it possible for you to nourish your diabetic child *and* the rest of your family. They reflect the principles of good nutrition already outlined. They are low in fat, sugar, and salt, and many are good sources of fiber. At the same time, they're high in flavor and eye appeal.

To make planning for your diabetic child as easy as possible, this section is organized by meals: breakfast, lunch, snacks, and dinner. I've found it saves time to be able to locate a number of appropriate choices for each meal in one spot. After Brennan was diagnosed as having diabetes, I started a loose-leaf notebook along the same lines, with individual sections for breakfast, lunch, snacks, and dinner, each containing menu ideas and some recipes. Each menu was based on Brennan's allowed exchanges. Of course, your own child will have his own diet plan, so this book can't provide precise menus for everyone, but it does offer a great variety of foods and recipes and some possible combinations of recipes to give you menu ideas.

At the beginning of each meal chapter are some general guidelines for concocting nutritious menus as well as specific tips on various foods or dishes commonly served at that meal and where they fit into the scheme of things for the diabetic. Your child's diabetes probably means that certain items will have to be cut from your shopping list, but I mention substitutes and alternatives wherever possible. The idea is to assist your child in learning about good nutrition and good diabetes management while making the restrictions imposed as painless as possible.

It's equally important that the job of planning and preparing your child's meals be trouble-free. Therefore, in the introductory pages of each chapter I've provided a full list of the recipes that follow, complete with their exchanges. Use it as an at-a-glance reference for designing your daily meals.

Please don't be limited by the way I've organized the recipes. Your child can certainly have leftover Spinach Manicotti for breakfast or a bowl of cereal for dinner. One of the problems with diabetes is that your child can't skip meals, no matter how much she dislikes what's on her plate. If you have a picky eater, you quickly learn the meaning of flexibility. Be as creative as you need to be in providing a finicky eater with healthy choices for meals and snacks. Toddlers can be especially difficult but will often respond to decorated foods or frozen treats like frozen bananas, frozen grapes, or homemade juice Popsicles.

At the end of the book, before the index, I've listed all the recipes by type—main dishes, desserts, vegetables, beverages, etc. This master list is meant to serve as an additional time-saver. Use it to formulate meals that correspond to your child's tastes and diet plan and that please and nourish your whole family.

Regarding servings, the best way to become familiar with the recommended portion for any exchange is to know what it looks like. For example, measure ½ cup of several different vegetables and see how much room is taken up on your child's plate. Compare a 3-ounce serving of meat, chicken, or fish to the size of your child's palm so she can see how big it is. For a week or two, weigh and measure everything and you and your child will get to a point where you can easily "eyeball" a serving and tell if it is about right. No one really expects you and your child to drag measuring cups and spoons and a scale around for the rest of your lives. Diabetes management is not a precise science. Food, exercise, and insulin requirements are a little different each day. The best we can hope for is a responsible approach and a fairly conscientious use of the tools we are given to help control blood sugar. Don't make yourself or your child crazy over one tablespoon more or less or ¼ FRUIT exchange; it's the overall picture that matters.

A NOTE ON SWEETNESS

Some of the recipes in this book do contain a small amount of sugar. The largest amount per serving is 1 teaspoon. There's nothing inherently wrong with a small amount of sugar when it's ingested with an otherwise wholesome food that contains fiber and some protein or fat. It's the concentrated sugars served in a food with no nutritional value that are detrimental to people with diabetes. Your child's blood sugar response to food is individualized; what raises one child's sugar greatly may not affect another child nearly as much. You and your child can judge by experience which foods are no-nos. If you have any questions, consult your doctor or dietician. Something like Wholesome Brownies (see index) may be fine for your child to have before a period of exercise when the NPH insulin is also peaking, but it may not be appropriate at other times. Timing of insulin and food intake can be important, and this subject is discussed in greater depth in Part III: "The Copebook."

Concerning artificial sweeteners, I have noted when it is appropriate to use Equal (aspartame). It is preferred because, thus far, it has been shown to be safe for human consumption and approved by the FDA. Its drawback is that it breaks down at the boiling point (212°F), so it cannot be used for baking. Saccharin (Sweet'n Low and SugarTwin), on the other hand, can be heated above the boiling point but has been identified as possibly carcinogenic.

Equal, Sweet'n Low, and SugarTwin come in standardized packets of approximately 1 gram by weight that are each equal in sweetness to 2 teaspoons of sugar. This is the size packet referred to in the recipes. Six of these packets would be equal in sweetness to ¼ cup sugar. If you like to buy SugarTwin in the pour-spout box, measure it just like sugar. I have given the comparative "sugar" sweetness of the artificial sweetener in each recipe. You can use that "sugar" amount as a guide when using SugarTwin.

As a parent, you need to make a decision as to how much artificial sweetener your child ingests each day. There is the previously discussed trade-off of good control and lessened risks of complications for the use of artificial foods with unknown long-term consequences. It is best for your child to eat whole, natural foods as much as possible, but your child is going to want to have some "sweets and treats" now and then. Your doctor and dietician or nurse-educator can help you with any specific questions that arise on this issue.

A NOTE ON INGREDIENTS

- All the fruits and juices used in these recipes are unsweetened. They can be fresh or canned in juice or water-packed. Remember that fruit juice contains carbohydrates and cannot be considered a free food for diabetics, so drain all canned fruits unless the recipe instructs otherwise.
- The baking powder used in the recipes should be double-acting. If you wish, you can get low-sodium baking powder in health food stores and double the amount listed to get the same effect.
- *Zest*, be it orange or lemon, refers to the colored portion of rind and does not include the white part underneath, which can be bitter.
- All the yogurt used in the recipes is plain, nonfat

yogurt. The buttermilk used should be made from skim milk. If you can't get it, get buttermilk made from low-fat milk and add 5 grams fat and 1 FAT exchange per cup used.

- All the herbs used should be dried leaves unless a recipe specifically states *ground* or *fresh*. Be sure to crush leaves in the palm of your hand or with a mortar and pestle to release the flavor before adding.
- Be sure to use fresh lemon juice. Reconstituted lemon and lime juices contain preservatives and just don't taste the same as fresh. The quality of ingredients is just as important as the recipe.
- *Don't* use garlic powder or garlic salt. Use fresh garlic. It's a wonder. Not only does it add distinctive flavor; it also is available year-round. More importantly, it possesses healthful properties far beyond just chasing vampires away. It can, in the right circumstances, lower serum cholesterol levels and triglyceride levels. Garlic and onions also contain substances that inhibit the clumping of blood cells. Clumping is the start of blood clots, which are a major factor in heart attacks and strokes.

  Choose heads of garlic that are plump, firm, dry, and free of soft or shriveled cloves. Store in a cool, dark, dry, well-ventilated spot, but not in the refrigerator, where it might sprout. Use lemon juice or salt to rid your hands or utensils of garlic odor. The chlorophyll in parsley helps freshen garlic breath.

This section was prepared under the expert guidance of Patty McCarthy and Tina Leeser. Patty, the mother of three hungry teenagers, is a gourmet chef who has studied in France. She and her mother have taught cooking classes for years in the southern California area under the name of "Cookworks." Tina closely supervised and guided the choice of recipes and provided all the nutrition and exchange information.

6
Breakfast

We've all heard that a good nutritious breakfast is important; for anyone with diabetes, it's essential. Of course, every meal is essential, but breakfast can present a special problem. Your child may not feel hungry first thing in the morning. He may simply refuse to eat his complete allotment of exchanges before leaving for school. You may have to resort to sending him off with some food in hand in the hope it will be eaten on the way to school. Your child may fail to do so, as happened when I tried this with Brennan. About halfway through the morning, I got a call from school. Brennan had had a severe insulin reaction and had to be carried to the school nurse. It helped him understand why breakfast was a good idea.

What is a good breakfast? Most of us with a diabetic person in the family have a pretty good idea. We've probably been told to include BREAD, FRUIT, and MILK exchanges and maybe a MEAT exchange or two. This meal is a perfect opportunity to fill your child with high-fiber, nourishing plant protein and fiber-filled fruit. Choosing whole grains and fresh fruits with low-fat milk products is the best approach.

Don't be limited by the standard breakfast fare of cereal with milk and fruit. My boys long ago got tired of cereal every morning. That's why I've included lots of muffin recipes along with recipes for sweet potato pie and bread pudding. Actually, you can serve anything that fits your child's diet plan for breakfast. The shakes included can be presented to a finicky eater as a special treat. You can also try many of the recipes in "Snacks," such as Baked

Custard, Brennan's Rice Pudding, and Apple Crunch. Maybe you'll find a few new favorites for your child, and you can alternate them with more traditional breakfast foods. If your child likes a food, and it's nutritious, serve it.

Think about breakfast the night before, even the weekend before. On Sunday night, make a batch of muffins and a big bowl of fresh fruit salad that will provide a few breakfasts and snacks. I often bake two sweet potato pies. One is used for dinner as a side dish, and one is for breakfast and snacks the next day. Homemade bread, baked the night before, can be a welcome treat the next morning.

As I've already stressed, it's the quality of food that is so important. Here are some guidelines that will help you make the best choices for breakfast.

- Choose skim (nonfat) or low-fat milk, yogurt, and buttermilk instead of whole milk and whole milk products.
- Serve whole, fresh, seasonal fruits as much as possible. Chunks of melon or orange wedges already on the breakfast table are usually eaten without much fuss. One piece of whole fruit usually will fill you up, but it's easy to drink the equivalent of several pieces of fruit as juice without realizing it.
- Get rid of bacon. It is high in fat and salt and has added sugar. It adds nothing to your family's health. Bacon and some other preserved meats are processed with sodium nitrate and sodium nitrite, which have been found in studies to be carcinogenic. Nitrates combine with the amines in the meat protein in your stomach to form nitrosamines. Nitrosamines have caused cancer in every animal species tested. Bacon is simply not worth it. If your family is used to it or some other form of meat in the morning, try homemade sausage or a plain hamburger patty instead (with wheat germ added for extra nutrition). If you must use it occasionally, use Canadian bacon or

pancetta, an Italian bacon available in Italian delis. Pancetta is cured with salt but without nitrates.

- Carbohydrates, ideally complex ones, are an important part of your breakfast menu. Remember, as a rule, the more processed a food, the less complex and more refined the carbohydrates. Refined carbohydrates generally cause the blood sugar to rise more quickly and to higher levels than complex ones containing more fiber. Also, the less refining, the more naturally occurring nutrients that will be present.

- A small amount of fat at each meal (1 FAT exchange or 1 teaspoon) helps delay the rise of blood sugar. This fat may be in muffins or pancakes or may be the margarine used on toast.

- Stay away from commercial granola and "natural" cereals. They have too much added fat and sugar. The sugar takes many forms—honey, brown sugar, corn syrup, and molasses. The fat is usually saturated vegetable fat, such as coconut or palm oil or hydrogenated soybean oil. Granola has less fiber than you would think, often less than Grape Nuts.

Be very careful about how you select the cereals you buy. As a general rule, the shorter the list of ingredients, the more nutritious the product. Look for a whole grain as the first listed ingredient, preferably with no added sugar or salt. Some good choices are:

> Nabisco's Spoon Size Shredded Wheat
> Oat Bran
> Wheatena
> Farina or Cream of Wheat
> Nutri-Grain, Wheat or Corn
> Wheaties
> Wheat Chex
> Total
> Puffed Wheat
> Quaker Oats—old-fashioned or quick-cooking

(don't use the instant; it's high in sodium
and sugar and has many additives)
Fortified Oat Flakes
Grape Nuts

Ingredients are listed on packages by order of weight. In other words, there's more of the first ingredient than anything else. Obviously, you won't buy a cereal that has sugar as the first ingredient. Check the "Carbohydrate Information" on the side of the box. Look for products that contain no more than 3 or 4 grams sucrose and other sugars (1 teaspoon of sugar weighs about 4 grams). Cereals with raisins or dates would show a higher sugar content, but it is provided by the fruit, which is high in nutrients and not just empty calories.

Most recommended serving portions of cereals appropriate for your diabetic are counted as 1½–2 BREAD exchanges, according to *The Diabetic's Brand-Name Food Exchange Handbook* by Andrea Barrett (Running Press, Philadelphia, 1984). That includes cereals with and without raisins and dates. Granola is higher in calories and counted as 1–1½ BREAD and ½–1½ FRUIT exchanges.

Also watch for sodium levels in cereals, as they can be very high. Reasonable amounts of sodium, less than 200 grams, are found in Nutri-Grain, All Bran, Most, Product 19, and Grape Nuts. Many hot cereals have less than 10 milligrams of sodium per serving, but adding only ⅛ teaspoon of salt per serving adds 275 milligrams. Try adding ⅛ teaspoon of cinnamon and a little artificial sweetener or a few chopped dates or raisins per serving instead of salt.

BREAKFAST MENU IDEAS

These will need to be altered to fit your child's diet plan, but they should give you some ideas. If you use low-fat (2-percent) milk versus skim milk, add 1 FAT per cup. If you use low-fat yogurt versus nonfat yogurt, add 1 FAT per cup. (Check the index to locate recipes.)

MENU 1

Strawberry Shake	⅔ FRUIT, 1 MILK, ½ FAT
Cinnamon Toast	1 BREAD, 1 FAT

TOTAL: 1 BREAD, ⅔ FRUIT, 1 MILK, 1½ FAT

MENU 2

Apple Spice Oatmeal	1½ BREAD, ½ FRUIT
8 ounces skim milk	1 MILK
½ orange, cut into wedges	½ FRUIT

TOTAL: 1½ BREAD, 1 FRUIT, 1 MILK

MENU 3

2 Orange Cottage Cheese Muffins	2 BREAD, 1 FAT
8 ounces skim milk	1 MILK
½ banana or 1 small apple	1 FRUIT

TOTAL: 2 BREAD, 1 FRUIT, 1 MILK, 1 FAT

MENU 4

½ cup Bread Pudding	1 BREAD, ½ MILK, 1 FAT
1 orange, cut into wedges	1 FRUIT
4 ounces skim milk	½ MILK

TOTAL: 1 BREAD, 1 FRUIT, 1 MILK, 1 FAT

MENU 5

1 wedge Robin's Favorite: Sweet Potato Pie	1½ BREAD, 1 FRUIT, ½ lean MEAT, 1 FAT
8 ounces skim milk	1 MILK

TOTAL: 1½ BREAD, 1 FRUIT, 1 MILK, ½ lean MEAT, 1 FAT

MENU 6

2 Multigrain Pancakes	1½ BREAD, 1 FAT
½ cup Blueberry Sauce	1 FRUIT
8 ounces skim milk	1 MILK

TOTAL: 1½ BREAD, 1 FRUIT, 1 MILK, 1 FAT

MENU 7

1 cup Ambrosia	1½ FRUIT, trace FAT
1 Homemade Sausage patty	1½ lean MEAT
1 Blueberry Muffin	1 BREAD, ½ FAT
8 ounces skim milk	1 MILK

TOTAL: 1 BREAD, 1½ FRUIT, 1 MILK, 1½ lean MEAT, ½ FAT

BREAKFAST EXCHANGES
(Per Serving)

Use this list as a quick reference when planning breakfast menus. A glance at the right-hand column should give you ideas of what to serve for certain exchanges called for in your child's diet plan. The recipes are listed here in the same order as they appear in the chapter.

Banana Shake	½ BREAD, 1 FRUIT, 1 MILK
Orange-Pineapple Shake	2 FRUIT, ⅓ MILK
Strawberry Shake	⅔ FRUIT, 1 MILK, ½ FAT
Homemade Cocoa Mix	½ MILK, ½ FAT
Berry Yogurt	½ FRUIT, ½ MILK, ½ FAT
Peach Yogurt	½ FRUIT, ½ MILK, ½ FAT
Ambrosia	1½ FRUIT, trace FAT
Spiced Baked Apples	2 FRUIT
Apple Spice Oatmeal	1½ BREAD, ½ FRUIT
Stovetop Granola	1 BREAD, 1 FAT
Homemade Sausage	1½ lean MEAT
Eggs Benedict	1 BREAD, 2 medium-fat MEAT
Mock Hollandaise Sauce	½ medium-fat MEAT
Bread Pudding	1 BREAD, ½ MILK, 1 FAT
Robin's Favorite: Sweet Potato Pie	1½ BREAD, 1 FRUIT, ½ lean MEAT, 1 FAT
Raisin Cheese Toast	1 BREAD, 1 medium-fat MEAT
Variation 3	1 BREAD, 1 FRUIT, 1 medium-fat MEAT

Cinnamon Toast	1 BREAD, 1 FAT
French Toast	1 BREAD, 1½ lean MEAT
Baked Apple Pancake	1 BREAD, 1 FRUIT, 1 medium-fat MEAT
Multigrain Pancakes	1½ BREAD, 1 FAT
Cheese Blintzes	1 BREAD, 2 medium-fat MEAT
Bran Crêpes	1 BREAD, 2 medium-fat MEAT
Strawberry Sauce	1 FRUIT/Less than ⅔ cup FREE
Mock Sour Cream	⅓ lean MEAT
Gloria's Corn Bread	1 BREAD, 1 FAT
Buttermilk Biscuits	⅔ BREAD, ½ FAT
Banana Bread	1 BREAD, 1 FRUIT, ½ FAT
High-Protein Three-Grain Bread	1½ BREAD
Whole Grain Irish Soda Bread	1½ BREAD, 1 FAT
Refrigerator Bran Muffins	1 BREAD, ½ FRUIT, 1 FAT
Applesauce Muffins	1 BREAD, 1 FRUIT, ½ FAT
Blueberry Muffins	1 BREAD, ½ FAT
Orange Cottage Cheese Muffins	1 BREAD, ½ FAT
Oat Bran Muffins	1 BREAD, ½ lean MEAT, 1 FAT
Lemon Muffins	1 BREAD, 1 FAT
Strawberry Jam	Up to ¼ cup FREE
Blueberry Jam Spread	Up to ¼ cup FREE
Microwave Peach Jam	Up to ½ cup FREE
Fresh Blueberry Sauce	Up to ¼ cup FREE
Applesauce	1¼ FRUIT

Recipes

BREAKFAST SHAKES AND BEVERAGES

When accompanied by a piece of high-protein toast, breakfast shakes are one of the quickest breakfasts to prepare. Shakes like this are appealing to many children because they remind them of ice cream shakes. They also break the monotony of a glass of milk and a piece of fruit. See also "Snacks" for other breakfast shake possibilities.

Banana Shake

½ banana, peeled
1 cup skim milk *or* ¾ cup skim milk and ¼ cup plain low-fat yogurt
2 tablespoons wheat germ
1 teaspoon vanilla extract

1. Put ½ banana in freezer the night before you plan to serve the shake.
2. Put all ingredients in a blender or food processor, blend until smooth, and serve.

Yield: 1 1¼-cup serving

Nutritive values per serving:	CAL	CHO (gm)	PRO (gm)	FAT (gm)
	155	28	9	0

Food exchanges per serving: ½ BREAD, 1 FRUIT, 1 MILK

Orange-Pineapple Shake

½ cup unsweetened orange juice
½ cup crushed pineapple, in juice
2 tablespoons instant nonfat dry milk
¼ teaspoon vanilla extract

Put all ingredients in a blender or food processor, blend
until smooth, and serve.

Yield: 1 1-cup serving

Nutritive values per serving:

	CAL	CHO (gm)	PRO (gm)	FAT (gm)
	107	24	3	0

Food exchanges per serving: 2 FRUIT, ⅓ MILK

Strawberry Shake

½ cup skim milk
½ cup plain low-fat yogurt
½ cup frozen unsweetened whole
   strawberries
½ teaspoon vanilla extract
1 packet artificial sweetener (Equal)

Put all ingredients in a blender or food processor, blend
until smooth, and serve.

Yield: 1 1½-cup serving

Nutritive values per serving:

	CAL	CHO (gm)	PRO (gm)	FAT (gm)
	106	19	8	2½

Food exchanges per serving: ⅔ FRUIT, 1 MILK, ½ FAT

Homemade Cocoa Mix

There are now several good sugar-free cocoa mixes on the market, but it is more economical to make your own with this recipe.

> ¾ cup cocoa (unsweetened)
> 1 quart instant nonfat dry milk
> 16 packets artificial sweetener (Equal)

1. Mix ingredients well and store in an airtight container in a moderately cool place.
2. Use 3 tablespoons mix plus 8 ounces of boiling water for each serving.

Yield: 24 8-ounce cups cocoa

Nutritive values per 8-ounce serving:	CAL	CHO (gm)	PRO (gm)	FAT (gm)
	65	5	4	4

Food exchanges per 8-ounce serving: ½ MILK, ½ FAT

FRUITY BREAKFAST TREATS
Berry Yogurt

½ cup blueberries, raspberries, or
  strawberries (fresh or frozen, unsweetened)
2 packets artificial sweetener (Equal)
¼ teaspoon vanilla extract
1 cup low-fat yogurt*

1. Wash blueberries; mash them with sweetener.
2. Stir vanilla into yogurt; fold in berries.
3. Chill in small container for several hours or overnight.

Yield: 2 ¾-cup servings

Nutritive values per ¾-cup serving:	CAL	CHO (gm)	PRO (gm)	FAT (gm)
	60	11	4	2½

Food exchanges per ¾-cup
serving: ½ FRUIT, ½ MILK, ½ FAT

---

*If you use nonfat yogurt, subtract ½ FAT.

Peach Yogurt

⅔ cup fresh peaches, pared and diced, or
  canned peaches in juice, drained
1 teaspoon fresh lemon juice
2 packets artificial sweetener (Equal)
¼ teaspoon ground mace or nutmeg
1 cup plain low-fat yogurt*

1. Slightly mash diced peaches with lemon juice, sweetener, and mace or nutmeg.
2. Stir in yogurt; blend well.
3. Chill in a covered container several hours or overnight.

Yield: 2 ¾-cup servings

Nutritive values per ¾-cup serving:	CAL	CHO (gm)	PRO (gm)	FAT (gm)
	64	12	4	2½

Food exchanges per ¾-cup
serving: ½ FRUIT, ½ MILK, ½ FAT

If you use nonfat yogurt, subtract ½ FAT.

Ambrosia

Fresh fruit salad is great for breakfast or anytime. Use any combination of fruit you like. Unsweetened coconut can be found at health food stores. If you can't find it, you can use sweetened coconut. It would add a few calories per serving but not change the exchange values.

> 2 small apples, sliced
> 2 medium grapefruit, peeled and sectioned
> 2 medium oranges, peeled and sectioned
> ½ cup unsweetened orange juice
> 2 tablespoons shredded coconut
> (unsweetened if available)
> Mint sprigs (optional)

1. Combine first 4 ingredients; cover and chill 1 hour.
2. Arrange fruit in individual serving dishes; sprinkle with coconut and garnish with mint if desired.

Yield: approximately 6 1-cup servings

Nutritive values per 1-cup serving:	CAL	CHO (gm)	PRO (gm)	FAT (gm)
	74	16	0	1

Food exchanges per 1-cup
serving: 1½ FRUIT, trace FAT

Spiced Baked Apples

4   medium cooking apples
½   cup water
1   teaspoon fresh lemon juice
    Ground cinnamon, mace, and nutmeg

1. Preheat oven to 375°F.
2. Core apples to within ½ inch of bottom, leaving an inch-wide cavity. Peel about a 1-inch strip of skin from stem end of each apple.
3. Arrange apples in an 8-inch square or 9-inch round baking pan. Combine water and lemon juice; pour over apples. Sprinkle a pinch of cinnamon, mace, and nutmeg on each apple.
4. Cover and bake for 50–60 minutes, until apples are tender. Or put in microwave on HIGH for 4–6 minutes, until apples are tender, turning dish about halfway through the cooking time.

Yield: 4 servings

Nutritive values per serving:	CAL	CHO (gm)	PRO (gm)	FAT (gm)
	80	20	0	0
Food exchanges per serving:	2 FRUIT			

CEREALS
Apple Spice Oatmeal

This is a much healthier version of the commercial instant oatmeal. It contains much less sodium and no sugar. Oatmeal has twice the protein content of corn or wheat flakes cereal.

2 cups water
1 cup rolled oats (regular or quick, not instant)
⅛ teaspoon salt, if desired
1 apple, peeled and chopped or grated
½ teaspoon ground cinnamon

1. In a heavy saucepan, combine the water, oats, salt, and apples. Bring to a boil, reduce heat, cover, and simmer for 5 minutes, stirring often.
2. Stir in cinnamon just before serving.

Variation
Substitute 3 dates, finely chopped, for the apple.

Yield: 3 ¾-cup servings

Nutritive values per ¾-cup serving:	CAL	CHO (gm)	PRO (gm)	FAT (gm)
	138	25	5	2

Food exchanges per ¾-cup serving: 1½ BREAD, ½ FRUIT

Stovetop Granola

This is much better for you than the commercial granolas. Try a ¼-cup serving sprinkled over other cereal or stirred into berry yogurt for extra flavor and nutrition. If you can't find unsweetened coconut, use sweetened.

1¼ cups oatmeal (old-fashioned, regular or quick, not instant)
⅓ cup chopped walnuts or chopped unsalted peanuts
¼ cup wheat germ
⅓ cup sesame seeds
⅓ cup shredded coconut (unsweetened if available)
¼ cup raisins
½ teaspoon ground cinnamon

1. Place the oatmeal and nuts in a large cast iron skillet over medium heat. Stir constantly for about 5 minutes.
2. Add the wheat germ, sesame seeds, and coconut. Stir occasionally for another 10 minutes.
3. Remove from the heat and let cool to room temperature.
4. Add the raisins and cinnamon and stir. Store in an airtight container.

Yield: 10 ¼-cup servings

Nutritive values per ¼-cup serving:	CAL	CHO (gm)	PRO (gm)	FAT (gm)
	111	11	4	7

Food exchanges per ¼-cup serving: 1 BREAD, 1 FAT

MEAT DISHES

Homemade Sausage

1 pound very lean ground beef
1 teaspoon sage
½ teaspoon thyme
½ teaspoon salt
1 teaspoon finely ground pepper

1. Mix all ingredients together thoroughly.
2. Shape into 8 patties.
3. Broil. If pan-frying, drain off the fat as it collects.
4. Drain patties on paper towels.

Yield: 8 patties

Nutritive values per 1-patty serving:	CAL	CHO (gm)	PRO (gm)	FAT (gm)
	85	0	10	5

Food exchanges per 1-patty
serving: 1½ lean MEAT

Eggs Benedict

½ teaspoon peanut oil
6 1-ounce slices Canadian bacon
6 poached eggs
3 English muffins, split and toasted
   Mock Hollandaise Sauce (recipe follows)

1. Wipe a large skillet with oil; place over medium heat until hot. Place Canadian bacon in skillet; cook 3 minutes on each side or until browned. Place on paper towels to drain.
2. Place 1 slice Canadian bacon and 1 poached egg on each muffin half; top each with 2 tablespoons Mock Hollandaise Sauce. Serve immediately.

Yield: 6 servings

Nutritive values per serving:	CAL	CHO (gm)	PRO (gm)	FAT (gm)
	232	15	17	11

Food exchanges per serving: 1 BREAD, 2 medium-fat MEAT

Mock Hollandaise Sauce

You can use low-fat instead of nonfat yogurt; it will add only a negligible amount of fat per serving:

> 1 egg yolk
> ½ cup nonfat yogurt
> 1 tablespoon fresh lemon juice
> ⅛ teaspoon freshly ground white pepper

1. Combine all ingredients in a small saucepan; stir with a wire whisk until smooth.
2. Cook mixture over low heat, stirring constantly, 3–4 minutes or until thoroughly heated. Serve warm. (The sauce can be reheated, if necessary, but *very slowly* over very low heat.)

Yield: ¾ cup

Nutritive values per 2-tablespoon serving:	CAL	CHO (gm)	PRO (gm)	FAT (gm)
	8	5	5	4

Food exchanges per 2-tablespoon serving:	½ medium-fat MEAT

PUDDING AND PIE FOR BREAKFAST

Bread Pudding

½ teaspoon vegetable oil
4 slices whole wheat bread, cubed
¼ cup golden raisins or currants
2 whole eggs
2 egg whites
1 12-ounce can evaporated skim milk
½ cup skim milk
6 packets artificial sweetener (equal to ¼ cup sugar)
½ teaspoon ground cinnamon
2 teaspoons vanilla extract
1 teaspoon finely grated lemon or orange zest

1. Preheat oven to 325°F.
2. Wipe a 1½-quart casserole with oil. Place bread in bottom of casserole. Scatter raisins on top.
3. Beat eggs and egg whites until foamy; mix in remaining ingredients.
4. Pour egg mixture over bread.
5. Place casserole in a shallow pan. Pour hot water to depth of 1 inch around casserole.
6. Bake 1 hour, until a knife inserted halfway between center and outside edge comes out clean.

Yield: 8 ½-cup servings

Nutritive values per ½-cup serving:	CAL	CHO (gm)	PRO (gm)	FAT (gm)
	145	16	9	5

Food exchanges per ½-cup serving:

1 BREAD, ½ MILK, 1 FAT

Robin's Favorite:
Sweet Potato Pie

*Robin, my younger son, is a fussy eater. This is one dish
that gets him excited about breakfast. I often make two
of these, one for dinner and one for breakfast the next
morning. They don't last long. I prefer to use yams
because the texture is smoother than that of sweet
potatoes. Instead of mixing this with a blender or food
processor, use a potato masher or food mill. The fiber
won't break down quite so much.*

- 1 egg white
- 2 whole eggs
- 3 medium sweet potatoes or yams, cooked and peeled
- 6 packets artificial sweetener (equal to ¼ cup sugar)
- 1 8-ounce can crushed pineapple in juice, undrained
- ¾ cup evaporated skim milk
- 1 teaspoon vanilla extract
- ¼ teaspoon each ground nutmeg, ginger, and cinnamon
- 1 unbaked 9-inch pie shell

1. Preheat oven to 425°F.
2. Beat egg white and eggs in food processor.
3. Mash sweet potatoes and combine with egg mixture.
4. Add remaining ingredients except pie shell and mix well to combine.
5. Pour into pie shell and bake for 10 minutes. Reduce heat to 325°F and bake another 45 minutes. A knife inserted in the center should come out relatively clean.

Yield: 8 servings

Nutritive values per serving:	CAL	CHO (gm)	PRO (gm)	FAT (gm)
	210	31	6	7

Food exchanges per serving: 1½ BREAD, 1 FRUIT, ½ lean MEAT, 1 FAT

TOAST, PANCAKES, AND MORE
Raisin Cheese Toast

¼ cup low-fat cottage cheese
1 packet artificial sweetener (Equal)
¼ teaspoon maple extract
   Dash ground nutmeg or cinnamon
1 slice whole wheat raisin bread, toasted

1. Combine the first 4 ingredients and spread on bread.
2. Place bread on foil or broiler pan and broil 6 inches from heat until cheese is hot and bubbly. Or use the toaster oven for the same result.

Variations
1. Use ½ English muffin instead of bread.
2. Substitute 2 tablespoons unsweetened orange juice and ½ teaspoon grated orange zest for maple extract and spices.
3. Omit maple extract, use ⅛ teaspoon ground cinnamon, and top with ½ banana, 1 peach, or 1 apple, sliced. Then broil as above.

Yield: 1 serving

Nutritive values per serving:	CAL	CHO (gm)	PRO (gm)	FAT (gm)
	150	19	7	5

Food exchanges per serving: 1 BREAD, 1 medium-fat MEAT

Nutritive values of Variation 2 per serving:	CAL	CHO (gm)	PRO (gm)	FAT (gm)
	160	19	7	5

Food exchanges of Variation 2 per serving: (exchanges unaffected)

Nutritive values of Variation 3 per serving:		CHO	PRO	FAT
	CAL	(gm)	(gm)	(gm)
	173	25	7	5

Food exchanges of Variation 3 per serving: 1 BREAD, 1 FRUIT, 1 medium-fat MEAT

Cinnamon Toast

Even the little ones can help make this!

> 1 slice high-fiber or high-protein whole wheat bread
> 1 teaspoon diet margarine
> Ground cinnamon
> 1 packet artificial sweetener (Equal)

1. Toast the bread.
2. Spread on the margarine, and sprinkle on the cinnamon and sweetener.

Yield: 1 serving

Nutritive values per serving:		CHO	PRO	FAT
	CAL	(gm)	(gm)	(gm)
	115	15	2	5

Food exchanges per serving: 1 BREAD, 1 FAT

French Toast

I like Nathan Pritikin's advice about cutting cholesterol whenever possible. Instead of using 2 whole eggs, I discard the yolk from one and cut down on the cholesterol. Try it for any egg recipe you use. Two egg whites equal one whole egg in volume.

1 egg white
1 whole egg
¼ cup skim milk
¼ teaspoon ground cinnamon
⅛ teaspoon ground nutmeg
½ teaspoon vanilla extract
4 slices whole wheat bread
½ teaspoon peanut oil

1. In a pie plate, mix all ingredients except bread and oil. Dip bread into mixture, one slice at a time, turning to coat both sides.
2. Wipe a nonstick griddle with the oil and heat over medium heat. Cook each side until golden.

Variation

Substitute ⅓ cup unsweetened orange juice for the milk and 1 teaspoon grated orange zest for the cinnamon.

Yield: 4 slices

Nutritive values per 1-slice serving:	CAL	CHO (gm)	PRO (gm)	FAT (gm)
	102	16	6	1

Food exchanges per 1-slice serving:

1 BREAD, 1½ lean MEAT

Baked Apple Pancake

This is a slight variation on a recipe from The Art of
Cooking for the Diabetic, *by Katharine Middleton and
Mary Abbott Hess (Contemporary Books, 1978).*

1 large cooking apple
½ cup skim milk
½ cup unbleached white flour
2 whole eggs, beaten
1 egg white
1 teaspoon sugar
½ teaspoon vanilla extract
Dash salt
2 tablespoons diet margarine
1 teaspoon ground cinnamon
4 packets artificial sweetener (Equal)
2 tablespoons fresh lemon juice

1. Preheat oven to 400°F.
2. Core apple and slice very thin.
3. Combine the skim milk, flour, eggs and egg white, sugar, vanilla, and salt. Mix until smooth. *Do not beat.*
4. Melt 1 tablespoon of the margarine in a 10-inch frying pan and "roll" it around so sides and bottom are covered. Add apple slices and sauté slightly.
5. Pour batter on top evenly. Bake in oven about 10 minutes or until pancake is puffy and nearly cooked. Sprinkle with cinnamon and sweetener, dot with remaining 1 tablespoon margarine, and return to oven to brown pancake.
6. Before serving, sprinkle with lemon juice. Cut in quarters to serve.

Yield: 4 servings

Nutritive values per serving:	CAL	CHO (gm)	PRO (gm)	FAT (gm)
	190	27	7	5

Food exchanges per serving: 1 BREAD, 1 FRUIT, 1 medium-fat MEAT

Multigrain Pancakes

These healthy goodies are from Jane Brody's Good Food Book. My kids said they were the best pancakes I ever made. Serve them with "lite" syrup or topped with sliced apples or pears sautéed in a little water in a nonstick pan with a generous sprinkling of cinnamon. (A note about "lite" syrups: they contain less sugar and can be counted as a FRUIT. For example, 2 tablespoons of Aunt Jemima Lite has 13 grams carbohydrate and would be 1⅓ FRUIT.) If you do not have oat flour or an alternative, simply add another ¼ cup of whole wheat flour to the dry-ingredients mixture.

Dry Ingredients
⅔ cup whole wheat flour, preferably stone-ground
⅓ cup unbleached white flour
¼ cup oat or other flour (e.g., cornmeal, barley, buckwheat, or millet flour)
2 tablespoons wheat germ
2 teaspoons sugar
1 teaspoon double-acting baking powder
½ teaspoon baking soda

Wet Ingredients
1 cup low-fat buttermilk
¼ cup or more skim milk
1 egg white
1 whole egg
1 tablespoon vegetable oil
¼ teaspoon vanilla extract (optional)

1. Mix together all the dry ingredients in a medium bowl.
2. In a second bowl, combine all the wet ingredients, whipping them enough to beat the egg white and the whole egg lightly. Add these to the dry ingredients, stirring just to combine them. The batter can stand for 10 minutes out of the refrigerator or for an hour or more refrigerated.

3. Heat the griddle over medium heat. Grease it lightly (if not nonstick) and immediately pour in ¼ cup batter. Try to leave some space between the pancakes to keep them from sticking together. Turn the heat down to moderately low and cook the pancakes until the bottoms are golden brown and the tops begin to bubble. Flip them over and cook them until the undersides are golden brown. Serve them immediately.

Yield: 12 pancakes

Nutritive values per 2-pancake serving:	CAL	CHO (gm)	PRO (gm)	FAT (gm)
	140	23	5	3

Food exchanges per 2-pancake serving:	1½ BREAD, 1 FAT

Cheese Blintzes

2 12-ounce cartons low-fat cottage cheese
1 egg, beaten
4 packets artificial sweetener (Equal)
1½ teaspoons grated lemon zest
¼ teaspoon vanilla extract
16 Bran Crêpes (recipe follows)
2 recipes Strawberry Sauce (recipe follows)
  Mock Sour Cream (optional) (recipe follows)

1. Preheat oven to 350°F.
2. Combine first 5 ingredients and stir well. Spoon about 3 tablespoons cheese filling in center of each blintz. Fold right and left sides over filling; then fold bottom and top over filling, forming a square.
3. Use a nonstick baking sheet. Place blintzes, seam side down, on baking sheet; bake for 12 minutes or until thoroughly heated.
4. Top each serving of 2 blintzes with ⅓ cup Strawberry Sauce. Serve with Mock Sour Cream if desired and add appropriate exchanges.

Yield: 16 blintzes

Nutritive values per 2-blintz serving (with filling and sauce):	CAL	CHO (gm)	PRO (gm)	FAT (gm)
	185	12	14	9

Food exchanges per 2-blintz serving (with filling and sauce): 1 BREAD, 2 medium-fat MEAT

Bran Crêpes

    3 eggs
    1½ cúps skim milk
    1 cup all-purpose flour
    ⅓ cup 100 percent bran cereal
    2 packets artificial sweetener (equal to 4
       teaspoons sugar)
    ¼ teaspoon salt
    2 teaspoons vegetable oil

1. Combine all ingredients except oil in container of a blender or food processor; process 30 seconds. Scrape down sides of blender container with a rubber spatula; process an additional 30 seconds or until smooth. Refrigerate batter 1 hour. (This allows flour particles to swell and soften so that crêpes are light in texture.)
2. Wipe the bottom of a 6-inch nonstick skillet with a bit of oil; place pan over medium heat until just hot, not smoking.
3. Pour about 2 tablespoons batter into pan. Quickly tilt pan in all directions so that batter covers the pan in a thick film; cook crêpe about 1 minute.
4. Lift edge of crêpe to test for doneness. Crêpe is ready for flipping when it can be shaken loose from pan. Flip the crêpe and cook for about 30 seconds. (This side is rarely more than spotty brown and is the side on which filling is placed).
5. When crêpe is done, place on a towel to cool. Repeat procedure until all batter is used, stirring batter occasionally. Stack crêpes between layers of waxed paper to prevent sticking.

Yield: 16 crêpes

Nutritive values per 2-crêpe serving:	CAL	CHO (gm)	PRO (gm)	FAT (gm)
	82	12	4	2

Food exchanges per 2-crêpe
serving: 1 BREAD, ½ FAT

Strawberry Sauce

This is good not only with blintzes but also with Vanilla Cheesecake (see index for recipe).

1½ cups fresh whole strawberries
1   packet artificial sweetener (Equal)
1   tablespoon fresh lemon juice

1. Wash berries and remove hulls and bad spots. Cut berries into bite-sized pieces.
2. Place in a bowl, crushing bottom layer slightly with a fork. Add sweetener and lemon juice and mix well.
3. Cover and chill.

Yield: 1⅓ cups

Nutritive values per ⅔-cup serving:	CAL	CHO (gm)	PRO (gm)	FAT (gm)
	40	10	0	0

Food exchanges per ⅔-cup serving: 1 FRUIT (up to ½ cup FREE)

Mock Sour Cream

Also use this on baked potatoes.

½   cup low-fat cottage cheese
1½ teaspoons fresh lemon juice

1. Combine all ingredients in container of a blender or food processor; process on medium-high speed until smooth and creamy.
2. Cover and chill thoroughly.

Yield: ½ cup

Nutritive values per 2-tablespoon serving:	CAL	CHO (gm)	PRO (gm)	FAT (gm)
	20	0	2	1

Food exchanges per 2-tablespoon serving: ⅓ lean MEAT

BREADS, BISCUITS, AND MUFFINS

Gloria's Corn Bread

I don't make this often because I could finish the whole pan myself—not to mention the difficulty of keeping Brennan from eating too much of it! It's filled with fiber that helps slow down the rise of blood sugar. That's important to your child.

> 1 cup unbleached white flour
> 1 cup stone-ground cornmeal
> ½ teaspoon salt
> 2 teaspoons double-acting baking powder
> ½ cup wheat germ
> 1 cup skim milk
> 2 tablespoons vegetable oil
> 3 packets artificial sweetener (equal to 2 tablespoons sugar)
> 1 whole egg
> 2 egg whites
> 1 cup fresh or frozen corn

1. Preheat oven to 400°F.
2. Combine flour, cornmeal, salt, baking powder, and wheat germ.
3. Add remaining ingredients and stir well.
4. Pour into well-greased 8- by 8-inch pan.
5. Bake 20–25 minutes.

Yield: 16 2-inch squares

Nutritive values per serving:	CAL	CHO (gm)	PRO (gm)	FAT (gm)
	105	18	4	2

Food exchanges per serving: 1 BREAD, 1 FAT

Buttermilk Biscuits

1½ cups unbleached white flour, sifted
½ cup whole wheat flour
2 teaspoons double-acting baking powder
½ teaspoon baking soda
½ teaspoon salt
1 tablespoon sugar
5 tablespoons diet margarine
¾ cup low-fat buttermilk

1. Preheat oven to 425°F.
2. Sift together dry ingredients.
3. Cut in margarine with a pastry blender or 2 knives.
4. Add buttermilk all at once; blend with a fork just until flour is moistened and dough pulls away from the side of the bowl.
5. Turn out onto a lightly floured board or wax paper. Knead lightly for 30 seconds.
6. Roll out to a thickness of ½ inch. Cut with a 2-inch round cutter. Place 1 inch apart on a baking sheet. Bake 12–15 minutes.

Yield: 16 2½-inch biscuits

Nutritive values per 1-biscuit serving:	CAL	CHO (gm)	PRO (gm)	FAT (gm)
	72	12	1	2

Food exchanges per 1-biscuit serving: ⅔ BREAD, ½ FAT

Banana Bread

1½ cups whole wheat pastry flour
½ teaspoon salt
2 teaspoons double-acting baking powder
1 cup broken walnuts or pecans (optional)*
1¼ cups mashed banana
3 tablespoons vegetable oil
¼ cup honey
½ cup wheat germ
Grated zest of ½ lemon
2 teaspoons butter

1. Preheat oven to 350°F.
2. Sift flour, salt, and baking powder together. Add nuts and mix well until coated with flour.
3. Add banana, oil, honey, wheat germ, and lemon zest. Mix just until ingredients are combined.
4. Butter 4½- by 9-inch loaf pan or use nonstick loaf pan. Batter will be stiff; spread evenly in pan. Bake for about 45 minutes.

Yield: 18 ½-inch slices

Nutritive values per ½-inch-thick slice serving:	CAL	CHO (gm)	PRO (gm)	FAT (gm)
	134	23	2	6

Food exchanges per ½-inch-thick slice serving:	1 BREAD, 1 FRUIT, ½ FAT

*If no nuts are used, subtract 36 calories, 4 grams of fat, and ½ FAT per slice.

High-Protein Three-Grain Bread

This wonderful recipe comes from Jane Brody's Good Food Book. *It looks like a lot of work, but it really isn't. It just takes several hours to rise while you do something else! Actual preparation time is 20–25 minutes. If you can't get soy flour, use whole wheat flour.*

2½ cups boiling water
1 cup rolled oats (regular or quick, not instant)
¾ cup nonfat dry milk
½ cup soy flour
¼ cup wheat germ
¼ cup honey
1 teaspoon salt
3 tablespoons vegetable oil
½ cup warm water (105–115°F)
2 packages (2 scant tablespoons) active dry yeast
1 tablespoon sugar
5½–6 cups whole wheat flour, preferably stone-ground

1. Preheat oven to 375°F.
2. In a very large bowl, combine the boiling water, oats, dry milk, soy flour, wheat germ, honey, salt, and oil. Cool the mixture to warm.
3. Place the warm water in a small bowl and add the yeast and sugar, stirring to dissolve them. Let the mixture stand for about 10 minutes or until the yeast starts to bubble.
4. Add the yeast mixture and 2½ cups of the whole wheat flour to the oat mixture. Beat this for 2 minutes and then add enough of the remaining flour to form a dough that is easy to handle.
5. Turn the dough out onto a lightly floured board and knead it for about 10 minutes or until it is smooth and elastic. Place the dough in a large greased bowl, turning the dough to coat the top. Cover the bowl with a

dish towel and let the dough rise in a warm draft-free
place until it has doubled in bulk, about 1½ hours.
6. Punch down the dough and divide in half. Flatten each
   half into a rectangle about 18 inches long and 8 inches
   wide. Starting from the short end, roll up each rectangle, pressing with your fingertips to seal the loaf as you
   go. Seal the ends and place each loaf in a greased loaf
   pan, about 9 by 5 by 3 inches. Cover the pans with a
   dish towel and let the loaves rise until they have
   doubled in bulk, about 1 hour.
7. Bake the bread for about 35–40 minutes or until the
   loaves sound hollow when tapped.

Yield: 2 loaves

Nutritive values per ½-inch-thick slice serving:	CAL	CHO (gm)	PRO (gm)	FAT (gm)
	113	21	4	1

Food exchanges per ½-inch-thick slice serving:		
	1½ BREAD	

Whole Grain Irish Soda Bread

I also serve this at dinner, and it's a big hit.

> 1¼ cups whole wheat flour
> 1½ cups unbleached white flour
> ¼ cup each wheat germ and brown sugar
> ½ teaspoon salt
> 2 teaspoons each baking soda and double-acting baking powder
> 1½ cups low-fat buttermilk
> 2 tablespoons diet margarine, melted
> ½ cup currants or raisins

1. Preheat oven to 375°F.
2. In a bowl, stir together all dry ingredients.
3. Stir in buttermilk and margarine until batter is blended but still lumpy.
4. Fold in currants or raisins.
5. Spoon batter into buttered and flour-dusted 8-inch round pan; do not smooth the surface.
6. Bake for 40–45 minutes or until a pick inserted in the center comes out clean. Cool bread in the pan for 10 minutes, then turn out on a wire rack. Serve warm, cooled, or sliced and toasted.

Yield: 1 8-inch round loaf (16 wedges)

Nutritive values per 1-wedge serving:	CAL	CHO (gm)	PRO (gm)	FAT (gm)
	121	23	3	2

Food exchanges per 1-wedge serving: 1½ BREAD, 1 FAT

Refrigerator Bran Muffins*

The sugar in this recipe adds up to only 1 teaspoon per muffin. More importantly, they're filled with fiber, which slows down the rise of blood sugar. The best news is that this batter will keep in your refrigerator, tightly covered,

---

*For all the muffin recipes, I prefer to use nonstick muffin pans. You may also use paper muffin cups, or if necessary, lightly greased pans.

for up to 4 weeks. You can bake muffins as you need
them so that they're always fresh.

    1 cup whole bran cereal, such as All Bran or
       Bran Buds
    1 cup boiling water
    ½ cup safflower oil
    ¼ cup light or dark brown sugar
    ¼ cup honey
    1 apple, grated
    2 carrots, grated
    2 eggs
    2 cups low-fat buttermilk
  2½ cups whole wheat flour
  2½ teaspoons baking soda
    ½ teaspoon salt
  1½ cups oatmeal (regular or quick, not
       instant)
    ½ cup wheat germ

1. In a 2- or 3-quart container with a cover, stir together the bran cereal and boiling water. Let stand for 10 minutes.
2. In another bowl, combine the oil, sugar, honey, apple, and carrots. Beat the eggs into the mixture. Mix in the buttermilk.
3. Combine the bran mixture and the oil mixture.
4. In another bowl, combine flour, baking soda, salt, oatmeal, and wheat germ. Slowly mix them into the bran mixture. Cover and refrigerate for several hours or overnight.
5. You can bake these muffins as needed in a 400°F oven for 20–25 minutes, until browned and a toothpick inserted in the center comes out clean.

Yield: 24 muffins

Nutritive values per 1-muffin serving:	CAL	CHO (gm)	PRO (gm)	FAT (gm)
	134	20	3.3	5

Food exchanges per 1-muffin
serving: 1 BREAD, ½ FRUIT, 1 FAT

Applesauce Muffins

Applesauce makes these muffins delectably moist without overloading them with fat.

> 1¼ cups unsweetened applesauce
> 1 large egg
> 2 tablespoons oil
> 2 tablespoons honey
> 1 cup whole wheat flour (regular or pastry)
> 1 cup unbleached white flour
> 2 teaspoons double-acting baking powder
> ¾ teaspoon baking soda
> ½ teaspoon ground cinnamon
> ¼ teaspoon ground nutmeg
> ¾ cup raisins

1. Preheat oven to 375°F.
2. In a large bowl, beat together the applesauce, egg, oil, and honey. Set the bowl aside.
3. In a medium bowl, combine the whole wheat and white flours, baking powder, baking soda, cinnamon, and nutmeg. Add this to the applesauce mixture, stirring just to moisten the dry ingredients. Stir in the raisins and divide the batter among 12 muffin cups.
4. Bake the muffins for 20 minutes.

Yield: 12 muffins

Nutritive values per 1-muffin serving:	CAL	CHO (gm)	PRO (gm)	FAT (gm)
	128	23	3	2

Food exchanges per 1-muffin
serving: 1 BREAD, 1 FRUIT, ½ FAT

Blueberry Muffins

Brennan loves these blueberry muffins.

2 cups whole wheat pastry flour
2 tablespoons sugar
1 tablespoon double-acting baking powder
¼ teaspoon ground cinnamon
¼ teaspoon ground nutmeg
1½ cups fresh or frozen blueberries, thawed and drained
1 cup unsweetened orange juice
¼ cup diet margarine, melted
1 whole egg
1 egg white
1 teaspoon grated orange zest

1. Preheat oven to 400°F.
2. Combine the first 5 ingredients in a large bowl. Fold in blueberries. Make a well in the center of the mixture.
3. Combine orange juice, margarine, egg, egg white, and orange zest. Add to the dry ingredients. Stir just until moistened.
4. Fill muffin cups ⅔ full. Bake for 20–25 minutes, until golden.

Yield: 16 muffins

Nutritive values per 1-muffin serving:	CAL	CHO (gm)	PRO (gm)	FAT (gm)
	88	16	2	2

Food exchanges per 1-muffin serving: 1 BREAD, ½ FAT

Orange Cottage Cheese Muffins

1½ cups unbleached white flour
½ cup buckwheat or whole wheat flour
1 cup yellow cornmeal (preferably stone-ground)
4½ teaspoons double-acting baking powder
¼ teaspoon salt
6 packets artificial sweetener (equal to ¼ cup sugar)
2 eggs
1 cup low-fat cottage cheese
¾ cup low-fat buttermilk
¼ cup fresh orange juice
2 teaspoons grated orange zest
⅓ cup oil
2 tablespoons raisins

1. Preheat oven to 400°F.
2. In a large bowl, combine the flours, cornmeal, baking powder, salt, and sweetener; mix well.
3. In a small bowl, beat eggs lightly; mix in the cottage cheese, buttermilk, orange juice, zest, oil, and raisins.
4. Make a well in the center of the flour mixture and add liquid ingredients all at once. Stir with a fork just enough to blend ingredients.
5. Fill muffin cups ⅔ full. Bake in a 400°F oven until golden brown, about 20 minutes.
6. Turn out of cups and serve hot or cool, or wrap airtight and refrigerate or freeze. To reheat muffins, wrap in foil and place in a 350°F oven for 15 minutes if chilled, 25 minutes if frozen.

Yield: 24 muffins

Nutritive values per 1-muffin serving:	CAL	CHO (gm)	PRO (gm)	FAT (gm)
	89	11	4	3

Food exchanges per 1-muffin serving: 1 BREAD, ½ FAT

Oat Bran Muffins

This recipe comes from the Oat Bran cereal box and is very good. Oat Bran is one hot cereal both my boys will eat, and its soluble fiber helps lower cholesterol in the blood. It also has the highest protein content of any plant protein other than soybeans.

- 2¼ cups Oat Bran cereal
- 2 tablespoons brown sugar
- ¼ cup chopped nuts
- ¼ cup golden raisins
- 1 tablespoon double-acting baking powder
- ½ teaspoon salt
- ¾ cup skim milk
- 2 eggs, beaten
- 2 tablespoons honey
- 2 tablespoons vegetable oil

1. Preheat oven to 425°F.
2. Combine cereal, brown sugar, nuts, raisins, baking powder, and salt.
3. Add milk, eggs, honey, and oil; mix just until dry ingredients are moistened.
4. Fill muffin cups ¾ full. Bake 15–17 minutes or until golden brown.

Yield: 12 muffins

Nutritive values per 1-muffin serving:	CAL	CHO (gm)	PRO (gm)	FAT (gm)
	123	18	5	5

Food exchanges per 1-muffin serving: 1 BREAD, ½ lean MEAT, 1 FAT

Lemon Muffins

1 cup unbleached white flour
1 cup whole wheat pastry flour
2 tablespoons sugar
½ teaspoon salt
⅔ cup skim milk
⅓ cup fresh lemon juice
1 teaspoon grated lemon zest
¼ cup vegetable oil
1 medium egg
2 tablespoons golden raisins

1. Preheat oven to 400°F.
2. Mix dry ingredients.
3. Combine remaining ingredients. Mix together with dry ingredients. Stir with fork. *Do not beat.* Batter will be lumpy.
4. Fill muffin cups ⅔ full. Bake 20–25 minutes.

Yield: 12 muffins

Nutritive values per 1-muffin serving:	CAL	CHO (gm)	PRO (gm)	FAT (gm)
	110	15	2	4

Food exchanges per 1-muffin serving: 1 BREAD, 1 FAT

JAMS AND FRUIT SAUCES
Strawberry Jam

1 envelope sugar-free strawberry-flavored
  gelatin
1 cup boiling water
2 cups sliced fresh strawberries
  Grated zest of 2 oranges
  Grated zest of 1 lemon

1. In a small heatproof bowl, combine gelatin and boiling
   water, stirring until gelatin is completely dissolved.
2. Stir in strawberries and grated orange and lemon zest.
3. Allow to cool, then pour into glass jar. Cover and chill
   at least 1 hour before serving.

Yield: 2 cups

Nutritive values per 1-tablespoon serving:	CAL	CHO (gm)	PRO (gm)	FAT (gm)
	3	0	0	0

Food exchanges per 1-tablespoon
serving: Up to ¼ cup FREE

Blueberry Jam Spread

1 teaspoon unflavored gelatin
¼ cup water
2 cups fresh or frozen blueberries
½ cup water
1 teaspoon fresh lemon juice
6 packets artificial sweetener (Equal)

1. Combine gelatin and ¼ cup water, stirring well. Set aside.
2. Combine blueberries, ½ cup water, and lemon juice in a medium saucepan. Bring to a boil, reduce heat, and simmer, uncovered, 8 minutes, stirring frequently.
3. Remove saucepan from heat and add gelatin, stirring well until gelatin is dissolved. Let cool for 10 minutes and stir in sweetener.
4. Cool to room temperature. Pour into glass jars and cover tightly. Chill 4–6 hours or until mixture is thoroughly chilled. Store in refrigerator for up to 1 month.

Yield: 2 cups

Nutritive values per 1-tablespoon serving:	CAL	CHO (gm)	PRO (gm)	FAT (gm)
	5	0	0	0

Food exchanges per 1-tablespoon serving: Up to ¼ cup FREE

Microwave Peach Jam

4 cups frozen, unsweetened sliced peaches, thawed
5 tablespoons powdered fruit pectin
1 tablespoon fresh lemon juice
¾ teaspoon ground mace
4 packets artificial sweetener (Equal)

1. Mash peaches with a potato masher.
2. Combine peaches with pectin, lemon juice, and mace in a deep 2-quart casserole.

3. Cover with casserole lid and microwave on HIGH for 2 minutes. Stir well.
4. Cover and microwave an additional 3–4 minutes.
5. Cool for 10 minutes and stir in sweetener. Pour into freezer containers; cover and freeze.
6. To serve, let jam thaw in refrigerator. Store jam in freezer up to 1 year or in refrigerator up to 1 month.

Yield: 2 cups

Nutritive values per 1-tablespoon serving:	CAL	CHO (gm)	PRO (gm)	FAT (gm)
	5	0	0	0

Food exchanges per 1-tablespoon serving: Up to ½ cup FREE

Fresh Blueberry Sauce

This is very good over pancakes, French toast, and waffles. Brennan especially likes it.

1 tablespoon cornstarch
½ cup water
1 tablespoon fresh lemon juice
¼ teaspoon ground mace
2 cups fresh blueberries
3 packets artificial sweetener (Equal)

1. Combine cornstarch, water, lemon juice, and mace in a small saucepan.
2. Add blueberries; bring to a boil. Reduce heat and simmer 1–2 minutes, stirring constantly, until clear and thickened. Stir in sweetener. Serve sauce warm over pancakes.

Yield: 2 cups

Nutritive values per ¼-cup serving:	CAL	CHO (gm)	PRO (gm)	FAT (gm)
	24	6	0	0

Food exchanges per ¼-cup serving: Up to ¼ cup FREE

Applesauce

You can buy unsweetened applesauce now, but there's nothing as good as homemade.

> 4 medium cooking apples (about 1½ pounds)
> ½ cup unsweetened apple juice
> ¼ teaspoon ground cinnamon
> ⅛ teaspoon ground nutmeg

1. Peel, core, and cut apples into wedges; combine apples and apple juice in a saucepan.
2. Cook, uncovered, over medium-low heat 10–15 minutes or until apples are tender, stirring occasionally to break up apples.
3. Stir in spices. Add more water, if needed, to achieve desired consistency. Serve warm or chilled.

Yield: 8 ⅓-cup servings

Nutritive values per ⅓-cup serving:	CAL	CHO (gm)	PRO (gm)	FAT (gm)
	48	12	0	0

Food exchanges per ⅓-cup serving: 1¼ FRUIT

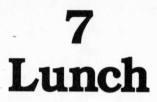

7
Lunch

Lunchtime for children with diabetes can be a dilemma for parents. Usually it boils down to whether to let your child eat the school lunch like most of his or her friends or take the old brown bag. It's a hard decision to make because there are so many variables. We've done a little of everything.

The most difficult part of school lunches is giving up complete control over the food your child is served. Especially if your child is newly diagnosed (the first year is the roughest), a natural fear and protectiveness can hold you in its power. When deciding how to handle lunch, keep a few things in mind:

Your child is a child first and a diabetic second. As much as is possible, it is very important to allow the child to lead a normal life, to be like "all the other kids." Diabetes is a train that takes you for a lifelong ride. The risk of controlling a child too tightly in childhood is that the child may get to her teens and say, "That's it. I've had enough of this diet-and-shot routine. Now I'll do it my way."

It is important to let your child take some responsibility for her diabetes as early as possible. That includes her making some bad choices now and then. If you're blood-testing, your child will be able to see the consequences of a poor choice, and you can discuss what might have been better. To apply that to lunch, your child might decide to eat the fruit salad served with the school lunch, not fully realizing that it's not the same as the apple you packed as a substitute. Her after-school blood sugar will tell the tale,

115

and she will understand next time. (By the way, she may still make the same choice. Only this time maybe she'll just eat a bite or two—just to be like the "other kids.")

You can formulate whatever plan suits your child's needs.

My son, Brennan, started by taking a lunch. First it was a lunch pail decorated with cartoon characters and a little thermos. As he got older, he started having the school lunch with everyone else because he didn't want to be different. Then we were able to get the monthly lunch menu, and I would send a bag lunch on days when the menu seemed inappropriate or it included something he didn't like. Lately he's been complaining about the food and wants to start taking his lunch again.

Getting a lunch menu plan from the school and going over it with your child gives you the broadest choice and helps both you and your child to think ahead. Simply mark off the lunches that seem inappropriate and plan to send a bag lunch on those days, as I did with Brennan.

Your child's brown bag or lunch box can be packed with anything from sandwiches to soups, stews, salads, and cut-up fresh vegetables and fruits. Brennan's current favorite lunch is a baked chicken breast with carrot sticks. You could add some homemade cookies and a piece of fruit to complete the exchanges. Little boxes of raisins are good for snacks to pack with lunch. Weight Watchers also makes dried apple snacks in foil pouches that are equal to one FRUIT.

The possibilities are endless when you have the right containers. Soups and stews stay steaming hot in those little individual-serving thermos jars. Tupperware makes a good lunch pail that has containers to hold sandwiches, drinks, anything moist like fruit salad, etc. Brennan likes to put a Tupperware glass of Crystal Light in the freezer overnight. The next morning he snaps the lid on, and by noon the drink has thawed but is still cold.

Any container with watertight, snap-on lids will work for the recipes in this chapter. However, some of these recipes won't do well sitting in a lunch pail for several hours. Tuna Melts, Mini Pizzas, and Sloppy Joes can be really unappealing if they're not served hot. They also get soggy after sitting around for a while.

Make a list with your child of all the brown bag possibilities and special favorites that will travel well. This gives your child a sense of control over his diet and gives you one place to look for menu possibilities. Make sure it includes choices for each of the exchanges in your child's lunch.

Now, about the recipes in this chapter. A wide selection of soups is included here because they can be made ahead and are very good for diabetics for several reasons. The soup recipes in this chapter are very low in fat and generally high in fiber. They give you more nutrition for fewer calories, and they are also filling. Soups containing vegetables are often eaten willingly by children who turn up their noses at the same vegetables presented on a dinner plate. Any of these soups can also be a good addition to dinner. Quite a few of them are almost a full meal of exchanges and make a satisfying main course accompanied by whole grain bread and fresh fruit for dessert.

It's much better to make homemade stock than to use canned. It's less expensive, for one thing, and you can make it almost totally fat-free and low in sodium. The easiest approach is to save leftover bones from chicken, turkey, and beef. (I find pork and lamb a little strong-flavored.) Have a bag in the freezer that holds the bones. Whenever it gets full, dump them into a pot and cover with water. Bring to a boil and then reduce heat to simmer. Add some cut-up onion, carrots, and celery. Simmer, covered, for a few hours. Let cool and place in the refrigerator. Skim all the fat that solidifies on the top. Strain the remaining broth and refrigerate. Freeze it if you won't be using it in a week or so.

You *can* use canned stock for the soup recipes that call for homemade stock. Try getting the new low-sodium stocks. Instead of adding extra salt, try adding fresh lemon juice or mild vinegar to any soup to give it extra zip.

Next, there are recipes for a few sandwiches, some main course dishes that adapt well to brown-bagging, and some salads. Macaroni and cheese and baked beans are good hot choices; pair them with cut-up vegetables and fruit. The potato salad and coleslaw are low-fat versions that you can use and season to your family's taste.

Most children have very strong opinions about the way sandwiches should be made, so it seemed presumptuous to include more than a few sandwich recipes. Sandwiches will, no doubt, be a mainstay of your child's homemade lunches, however, so the list below shows calories and exchanges for some common sandwich fillings. This is not by any means a complete list. Choose luncheon meats that emphasize 90–95 percent fat-free, preferably made from chicken or turkey. Try not to use only store-bought cold cuts for sandwiches. They're high in salt, sometimes have added sugar, and some are preserved with nitrates. Home-cooked chicken or turkey breast makes a great sandwich. Unsalted peanut butter is now available in many supermarkets. Try it. Your child probably won't notice the difference. For further reference, I highly rec- ommend *The Diabetic's Brand-Name Food Exchange Handbook*, by Andrea Barrett (Running Press, Philadel- phia, 1984).

SANDWICH FILLINGS

TUNA: Solid White in Water
½ can (3½ ounces)   120 calories/2 lean MEAT

TUNA: Chunk Light in Water
½ can (3½ ounces)   120 calories/2 lean MEAT

TURKEY: Luncheon Meat or Turkey Sausage
Louis Rich (1 slice)   40–60 calories/½ lean MEAT,
                              ½ FAT

HAM
Oscar Mayer 95% FAT FREE   25 calories/½ lean MEAT
  (1 slice)

SALAMI
Hebrew National beef, sliced   90 calories/½ lean MEAT, 1½ FAT
   (1 ounce)

CHICKEN
Weaver white-meat roll   40 calories/½ lean MEAT
   (1 ounce)

PEANUT BUTTER
Smuckers Natural   200 calories/1 lean MEAT, 3 FAT
   (2 tablespoons)

JAM
Smuckers Low Sugar   32 calories/1 FRUIT
   Strawberry or Grape Jam
   (4 teaspoons)

CHEESE
American, Monterey Jack, or   110 calories/1 lean MEAT, 1 FAT
   Swiss (1 ounce)

FRANKFURTERS: The best choices, if you must serve them, are
   chicken and turkey franks. All wieners and franks are very high in
   sodium.
Weaver Chicken (1 frank)   120 calories/1 lean MEAT, 1½ FAT
Louis Rich Turkey (1 frank)   100 calories/1 lean MEAT, 1 FAT
(All the beef franks have 2–3½ FAT exchanges per frank.)

LUNCH MENU IDEAS

These will need to be altered to fit your child's diet plan,
but they should give you some ideas. (Check the index to
locate recipes.)

MENU 1

Corn Chowder   2 BREAD, ½ medium-fat MEAT
8 ounces skim milk   1 MILK
Carrot and celery sticks   1 or 2 VEGETABLE
   (as much as desired)
⅔ cup strawberries   1 FRUIT

TOTAL: 2 BREAD, 1 FRUIT, 1 MILK, ½ medium-fat MEAT, 1–2
   VEGETABLE

MENU 2

Minestrone	3 BREAD, 1 lean MEAT
8 ounces skim milk	1 MILK
1 piece fruit or small box	1 FRUIT
raisins (2 tablespoons)	

TOTAL: 3 BREAD, 1 FRUIT, 1 MILK, 1 lean MEAT

MENU 3

2 Mini Pizzas	2 BREAD, 3 medium-fat MEAT, 1 VEGETABLE
½ Stuffed Baked Apple (from Breakfast chapter)	1 FRUIT
Carrot and celery sticks (as much as desired)	1 or 2 VEGETABLE

TOTAL: 2 BREAD, 1 FRUIT, 3 medium-fat MEAT, 2–3 VEGETABLE

MENU 4

1 Open-Faced Tuna Melt	1 BREAD, 3 lean MEAT
½ cup Coleslaw or	½ VEGETABLE, trace FAT
Special Fruited Coleslaw	½ FRUIT, 1 VEGETABLE
1 orange	1 FRUIT
8 ounces skim milk	1 MILK
1 Oatmeal Cookie (from Snack chapter)	½ BREAD, ½ FAT

TOTAL: 1½ BREAD, 1–1½ FRUIT, 1 MILK, 3 lean MEAT, ½–1 VEGETABLE, ½ FAT

MENU 5

Vegetable Soup (1⅓ cups)	1 BREAD, 2 VEGETABLE
1 Pita Pocket	1 BREAD, 2 lean MEAT, 1 VEGETABLE
Fruit salad (homemade) (½ cup of any fruit combination)	1 FRUIT
8 ounces skim milk	1 MILK

TOTAL: 2 BREAD, 1 FRUIT, 1 MILK, 2 lean MEAT, 3 VEGETABLE

LUNCH EXCHANGES

Use this list as a quick reference when planning lunch menus. A glance at the right-hand column should give you

ideas of what to serve for certain exchanges called for in
your child's diet plan. The recipes are listed here in the
same order as they appear in the chapter.

Egg Drop Soup	Up to 2 cups FREE
Minestrone	3 BREAD, 1 lean MEAT
Navy Bean Soup	1 BREAD, 1 lean MEAT, 1 VEGETABLE
Matzo Ball Soup	2 lean MEAT, 1 VEGETABLE
Matzo Balls	½ BREAD
Manhattan Clam Chowder	½ BREAD, 1½ lean MEAT, 1 VEGETABLE
Corn Chowder	2 BREAD, ½ medium-fat MEAT
Vegetable-Beef Soup	2 BREAD
Split Pea Soup	1 BREAD, 1 lean MEAT, 1 VEGETABLE
Vegetable Soup	1 BREAD, 2 VEGETABLE
Lentil Soup	1 BREAD, 3 VEGETABLE
Potato and Turnip Soup	½ BREAD, 2 VEGETABLE
Greek Lemon Soup	½ lean MEAT
Open-Faced Tuna Melts	1 BREAD, 3 lean MEAT, 1 VEGETABLE
Pita Pockets	1 BREAD, 2 lean MEAT, 1 VEGETABLE
Mini Pizzas	1 BREAD, 1½ medium-fat MEAT
Sloppy Joes	1 BREAD, 2 lean MEAT, 1 VEGETABLE
Baked Macaroni and Cheese	1 BREAD, 1½ medium-fat MEAT
Baked Beans	1 BREAD, ½ lean MEAT, 1 VEGETABLE
Turkey Chili	1 BREAD, 3 lean MEAT, 1 VEGETABLE
Chili Deluxe with Vegetables	1 BREAD, 2 lean MEAT, 2 VEGETABLE
New Potato Salad	1½ BREAD, 1 FAT
German Potato Salad	1 BREAD, 1 VEGETABLE, ½ FAT
Coleslaw	1 VEGETABLE, trace FAT
Special Fruited Coleslaw	1 FRUIT, 2 VEGETABLE

Recipes

SOUPS

Egg Drop Soup

This soup is good for lunch with a sandwich or good before a Chinese-style dinner entree like Beef and Snow Peas (see index for recipe).

> 4 cups homemade chicken stock
> ¼ cup sliced green onion (¼-inch pieces)
> 1 whole egg
> 1 egg white, slightly beaten
> 1 teaspoon soy sauce

1. Bring chicken stock to boil in a large saucepan. Add onions.
2. Remove from heat; slowly pour in egg and egg white, stirring gently as you pour. Add soy sauce and serve.

Variations
1. Add peeled, thinly sliced fresh gingerroot for extra stock flavor, but caution everyone not to eat it—it's *hot!*
2. If you like, you can thicken the soup slightly with 2 teaspoons cornstarch mixed with 2 tablespoons cold water stirred into the boiling stock in step 1.

Yield: 6 ⅔-cup servings

Nutritive values per ⅔-cup serving:	CAL	CHO (gm)	PRO (gm)	FAT (gm)
	15	0	2	1

Food exchanges per ⅔-cup serving: Up to 3 servings (2 cups) FREE

Minestrone

An easy way to half-cook the beans for this recipe is to put ½ cup (dried) of each in a large pot and cover with water. Bring to a boil and then simmer for 30 minutes, adding more water if necessary. You can use any stock for this, though beef stock is traditional.

2 quarts homemade stock
½ cup white wine
1 large onion, sliced thin
1 medium leek, sliced fine
2 cloves garlic, minced
2 medium carrots, sliced
2 medium unpeeled potatoes, cubed
1 green pepper, chopped
1 cup half-cooked dried navy beans
1 cup half-cooked dried garbanzos
1 cup half-cooked dried split peas
1 cup half-cooked dried lima beans
½ cup dried lentils
1 teaspoon oregano leaves
2 teaspoons basil leaves
1 teaspoon thyme leaves
1 bay leaf
Dash cayenne pepper
1 teaspoon ground cumin
Juice of 1 lemon
1 cup whole wheat elbow macaroni
1 cup green beans, cut into 1-inch pieces
2 small zucchini, sliced
1 cup chopped tomatoes (preferably fresh)
1 cup tomato puree
Grated Parmesan cheese

1. Bring stock and wine to a boil in a large soup pot. Add onion, leek, garlic, carrots, potatoes, green pepper, navy beans, garbanzos, peas, lima beans, lentils, seasonings, and lemon juice. Cover and simmer for 30 minutes or until vegetables are very soft but still holding their shape.

2. Add macaroni and cook for five minutes.
3. Add green beans, zucchini, tomatoes, and puree and cook for another 10 minutes or until macaroni is tender. To serve, sprinkle with a little grated Parmesan cheese.

Yield: 8 2-cup servings

Nutritive values per 2-cup serving:	CAL	CHO (gm)	PRO (gm)	FAT (gm)
	261	49	14	1

Food exchanges per 2-cup serving: 3 BREAD, 1 lean MEAT

Navy Bean Soup

1 cup each finely diced carrots and celery
½ onion, minced
1 clove garlic, minced
3½ cups water
1 cup tomato puree
1½ cups cooked navy beans
⅛ teaspoon freshly ground pepper
2 tablespoons chopped fresh parsley
¼ cup Parmesan cheese

1. In a 2-quart saucepan, combine carrots, celery, onion, garlic, water, and tomato puree and bring to a boil. Reduce heat and simmer until vegetables are tender, about 15 minutes.
2. Add beans, pepper, and parsley. Heat about 5 minutes longer. Sprinkle 2 teaspoons of cheese on each serving.

Yield: 6 1¼-cup servings

Nutritive values per 1¼-cup serving:	CAL	CHO (gm)	PRO (gm)	FAT (gm)
	130	20	8	2

Food exchanges per 1¼-cup serving: 1 BREAD, 1 lean MEAT, 1 VEGETABLE

Matzo Ball Soup

I love Matzo Ball Soup and so do my boys.

> 1 chicken, about 4 pounds
> 2 quarts water
> 1 whole onion, peeled and quartered
> 2 carrots, sliced
> 4 stalks celery, including tops, coarsely chopped
> Juice of ½ lemon
> 2 sprigs fresh parsley
> 2 sprigs fresh dill
> ¼ teaspoon freshly ground pepper
> 1 teaspoon salt
> Matzo Balls (recipe follows)

1. Clean the chicken and place it in a deep soup pot. Add water and the remaining ingredients except Matzo Balls. Bring to a boil, then simmer, covered, until the chicken is tender, about 2 hours. Remove the chicken, strain the soup, and chill.

2. Skim off the fat that rises to the top of the chilled soup. Reserve the cooked chicken for other recipes, like Chinese Chicken Salad. Reheat soup and add Matzo Balls, cooking as directed in recipe.

Yield: 8 1-cup servings

Nutritive values per 1-cup serving:	CAL	CHO (gm)	PRO (gm)	FAT (gm)
	103	4	13	4

Food exchanges per 1-cup serving:　　　　2 lean MEAT, 1 VEGETABLE

Matzo Balls

1   whole egg
2   egg whites
½   cup matzo meal
2   tablespoons finely minced onions
½   teaspoon ground cinnamon (optional)
1   tablespoon chopped fresh parsley
½   teaspoon salt (optional)
¼   teaspoon freshly ground white pepper
    Mixture of a little oil and water to lubricate
    hands

1. Beat the egg and egg whites. Fold in the matzo meal
    and seasonings; put mixture in refrigerator for 1 hour.
2. Mix a little oil and water to lubricate hands for forming
    balls. Form balls slightly larger than walnuts. Drop
    balls gently into boiling stock. Cover pot. Let simmer
    for 30 minutes. Remove from heat and let stand for 30
    minutes.

Yield: 10 medium-sized balls

Nutritive values per matzo ball:		CHO (gm)	PRO (gm)	FAT (gm)
	CAL			
	37	5	2	1

Food exchanges per matzo ball: ½ BREAD

Manhattan Clam Chowder

1 tablespoon diet margarine
1 cup diced onions
8 ounces potatoes, cut into cubes
1 16-ounce can tomatoes
2 cups diced carrots
1 green pepper, chopped
2 cups bottled clam juice
1 cup diced celery
1 cup water
1 teaspoon thyme leaves
Dash freshly ground pepper
2 10-ounce cans clams, drained
2 tablespoons or more chopped fresh parsley

1. In 4-quart saucepan, heat margarine until bubbly; add onions and cook until onions are translucent.
2. Add remaining ingredients except clams and parsley and bring to a boil. Reduce heat and simmer for 1 hour.
3. Add chopped clams and parsley and bring to a boil. Reduce heat and simmer 5 minutes longer.

Yield: 8 1½-cup servings

Nutritive values per 1½-cup serving:	CAL	CHO (gm)	PRO (gm)	FAT (gm)
	133	12	15	3

Food exchanges per 1½-cup serving:

½ BREAD, 1½ lean MEAT, 1 VEGETABLE

Corn Chowder

   2 tablespoons diet margarine
   1 small onion, minced
  ½ cup minced celery
   1 tablespoon all-purpose flour
  2¼ cups skim milk
   2 10-ounce bags frozen corn
  ¼ teaspoon salt
  ¼ teaspoon ground white pepper
  ⅛ teaspoon ground thyme
     Paprika

1. Melt margarine in a heavy 2-quart saucepan over medium heat; add onion and celery and sauté 5 minutes or until tender.
2. Stir in flour; cook over low heat 1 minute, stirring constantly.
3. Gradually add milk; cook over medium heat, stirring constantly, until thickened and bubbly. Stir in corn, salt, pepper, and thyme; simmer 20 minutes, stirring occasionally.
4. Just before serving, puree half the soup in blender or food processor. Return to saucepan and mix with remaining soup. To serve, ladle soup into bowls and sprinkle with paprika.

Yield: 4 1¼-cup servings

Nutritive values per 1¼-cup serving:	CAL	CHO (gm)	PRO (gm)	FAT (gm)
	191	33	8	3

Food exchanges per 1¼-cup serving:	2 BREAD, ½ medium-fat MEAT

Vegetable-Beef Soup

1 cup dried northern beans
1 cup dried split peas
3 quarts water
1 soup bone, split
2 large stalks celery, chopped
½ bunch fresh parsley, chopped
2 cloves garlic, diced fine
2 medium onions, chopped
2 medium potatoes, chopped
2 large carrots, sliced
1 large turnip, chopped
2 bay leaves
1 cup tomato puree
½ cup diced green pepper
½ cup diced sweet red pepper
1 cup cut-up fresh or frozen green beans
8 ounces broad noodles, broken into pieces
Paprika
1 teaspoon oregano
½ teaspoon rosemary
Dash Worcestershire sauce

1. Place beans and peas in bowl and add water to cover. Soak overnight. Drain.
2. Bring 3 quarts water to boil in stockpot. Add soup bone and simmer, covered, 3 hours. Remove soup bone.
3. To broth add drained beans and split peas, celery, parsley garlic, onions, potatoes, carrots, turnip, bay leaves, and tomato puree. Simmer, covered, about 2 hours or until legumes are tender. Add green and red pepper and green beans and cook 10–15 minutes, until tender. Add noodles and cook about 7 minutes or until noodles are tender. Add paprika to taste, oregano, rosemary, and Worcestershire. Remove bay leaves before serving.

Yield: 12 1-cup servings

Nutritive values per 1-cup serving:	CAL	CHO (gm)	PRO (gm)	FAT (gm)
	137	26	6	1

Food exchanges per 1-cup
serving: 2 BREAD

Split Pea Soup

8 ounces dried split peas
4 cups water
¾ cup chopped onion
½ cup chopped carrots
½ cup chopped lean ham
½ teaspoon ground celery seeds
¼ teaspoon salt
¼ teaspoon freshly ground pepper
¼ teaspoon marjoram leaves
⅛ teaspoon thyme leaves

1. Sort and wash peas; place in a Dutch oven. Add remaining ingredients and bring to a boil. Cover, reduce heat, and simmer 1 hour or until peas are tender.
2. Pour half of mixture into container of an electric blender or a food processor; process until smooth. Repeat with remaining mixture. Serve hot.

Yield: 6 1-cup servings

Nutritive values per 1-cup serving:	CAL	CHO (gm)	PRO (gm)	FAT (gm)
	157	25	12	1

Food exchanges per 1-cup
serving: 1 BREAD, 1 lean MEAT,
                                      1 VEGETABLE

Vegetable Soup

If you substitute canned stock, omit the salt.

> 4   cups homemade chicken, beef, vegetable, or turkey stock
> 1   16-ounce can tomatoes
> ½   cup chopped onions
> ½   cup thinly sliced carrots
> ½   cup diagonally sliced celery
> ½   cup coarsely chopped green pepper
> ½   teaspoon salt
> 2   tablespoons fresh lemon juice
> 5   whole peppercorns
> ½   teaspoon basil leaves
> ¼   teaspoon hot pepper sauce
> ½   cup alphabet pasta or any other small pasta, uncooked

1. Combine all ingredients except pasta in a 3- to 4-quart pot. Bring to a boil. Cover and simmer gently for 1 hour. Stir occasionally to break up tomatoes into bite-sized pieces.

2. Add pasta and cook for 5–7 minutes, until done.

Yield: 7 cups (5½ servings)

Nutritive values per 1⅓-cup serving:	CAL	CHO (gm)	PRO (gm)	FAT (gm)
	116	24	5	0

Food exchanges per 1⅓-cup serving: 1 BREAD, 2 VEGETABLE

Lentil Soup

4 cups homemade chicken stock
2 cups water
¼ cup red wine
1 cup dried lentils
½ cup long-grain brown rice
1 16-ounce can tomatoes, chopped
1 bay leaf
¼ cup chopped fresh parsley
1 teaspoon ground cumin
1 carrot, sliced
1 onion, chopped
1 celery stalk, sliced
2 garlic cloves, minced or pressed
Juice of ½ lemon
1 bunch (6–8 ounces) fresh spinach, cleaned and stemmed

1. Combine all ingredients except spinach in a 3- to 4-quart saucepan and bring to a boil. Reduce heat and cover. Simmer for 20–25 minutes or until lentils and rice are tender.
2. Cut spinach across the leaves in long, thin shreds. Add to soup and simmer for 5 minutes. Remove bay leaf and serve.

Yield: Approximately 8 1-cup servings

Nutritive values per approximate 1-cup serving:	CAL	CHO (gm)	PRO (gm)	FAT (gm)
	144	27	9	0

Food exchanges per approximate
1-cup serving: 1 BREAD, 3 VEGETABLE

Potato and Turnip Soup

This low-fat, hearty soup is from Jane Brody's Good Food Book.

  1 small onion, sliced thin (¼ cup)
  2 small white turnips (about ⅓ pound), peeled and sliced thin
  1 pound potatoes (about 3 medium), peeled and sliced thin
  3 cups homemade chicken broth
  1 cup skim milk
  ½ teaspoon ground nutmeg
     Freshly ground pepper to taste
  ¼ cup evaporated skim milk

1. In a large saucepan, combine the onion, turnips, potatoes, and broth. Bring the soup to a boil, reduce the heat, partially cover the pan, and simmer the soup until the vegetables are tender, about 10 minutes.
2. Transfer the vegetables and cooking liquid to a blender or food processor (in batches, if necessary) and puree them.
3. Just before serving, return the puree to a saucepan and heat the puree over a moderately low flame. Add the skim milk, nutmeg, and pepper and heat the soup to just below boiling. Stir in the evaporated milk and serve.

Yield: 6 1-cup servings

Nutritive values per 1-cup serving:	CAL	CHO (gm)	PRO (gm)	FAT (gm)
	84	17	4	0

Food exchanges per 1-cup serving:　　　½ BREAD, 2 VEGETABLE

Greek Lemon Soup

Here's the Greek version of egg drop soup, with the added tang of lemon and herbs.

> 4 cups homemade chicken stock
> 2 tablespoons long-grain rice
> 1 whole egg, beaten
> 1 egg white, beaten
> 2 tablespoons fresh lemon juice
> 1 tablespoon chopped fresh parsley
> ½ teaspoon oregano leaves
> Dash freshly ground black pepper

1. Bring stock to a boil. Add rice, cover, and turn heat down to simmer for 15–20 minutes, until rice is tender.

2. Mix egg, egg white, and lemon juice. Slowly pour egg mixture into stock, stirring gently, and simmer for 2–3 minutes.

3. Add herbs and pepper. Serve.

Yield: 4 servings

Nutritive values per 1-cup serving:	CAL	CHO (gm)	PRO (gm)	FAT (gm)
	32	3	4	1

Food exchanges per 1-cup
serving: ½ lean MEAT

SANDWICHES

For exchange information on some common sandwich fillings, refer to the list in the introduction to this chapter.

Open-Faced Tuna Melts

1   7-ounce can tuna, packed in water
2   tablespoons diet mayonnaise
2   tablespoons fresh lemon juice
2   tablespoons low-fat cottage cheese
2   teaspoons Dijon mustard
2   tablespoons finely minced red onion (optional)
4   slices whole grain bread, toasted
4   slices fresh tomato (optional)
$\frac{1}{2}$ cup grated American or Cheddar cheese

1. Drain tuna. Flake with a fork.
2. Combine next 5 ingredients and mix into tuna.
3. Spoon equal amounts on each slice of bread. Top with tomato and 2 tablespoons cheese each. Broil in toaster oven or broiler until cheese bubbles.

Yield: 4 servings

Nutritive values per serving:	CAL	CHO (gm)	PRO (gm)	FAT (gm)
	212	16	19	8

Food exchanges per serving: 1 BREAD, 3 lean MEAT

Pita Pockets

Pita bread comes in a whole wheat variety that is tasty and nutritious. Each round can be cut in half and filled like a little pocket—a nice change from regular sand- wiches. You can use turkey, tuna, or ground beef instead of the chicken listed here. Pita pockets can also hold the same ingredients used for tacos with much less mess.

- ½ pound cooked shredded chicken
- 2 tablespoons diced red onion
- ½ cup diced celery
- ½ green or red sweet pepper, diced
- 1 tablespoon diet mayonnaise
- 2 tablespoons plain nonfat yogurt
- 2 teaspoons fresh lemon or lime juice
- 1 teaspoon Dijon mustard
- Pinch cayenne pepper
- 2 pita rounds
- Shredded lettuce and alfalfa sprouts (optional)

1. Mix first 9 ingredients. Refrigerate for 30 minutes or longer.
2. Cut pitas in half and fill each pocket with one-quarter of the chicken mixture. Add a little lettuce or alfalfa sprouts if desired.

Yield: 4 pocket sandwiches

Nutritive values per serving:	CAL	CHO (gm)	PRO (gm)	FAT (gm)
	189	18	18	5

Food exchanges per serving:	1 BREAD, 2 lean MEAT, 1 VEGETABLE

Mini Pizzas

I normally don't serve frankfurters because they contain preservatives, but kids do like them. If you prefer not to serve them, make the pizzas without them and subtract ½ medium-fat MEAT exchange.

> 4 English muffins, split
> 1 8-ounce can tomato sauce
>   Dried oregano and dried basil
> 4 turkey frankfurters, sliced
> 8 teaspoons Parmesan cheese
> 8 slices (¼-inch thick) part-skim mozzarella cheese

1. Spread each muffin half with 2 tablespoons tomato sauce. Top with a pinch each of oregano and basil.
2. Put sliced ½ frankfurter onto each muffin. Top with 1 teaspoon Parmesan cheese and 1 slice mozzarella. Toast under broiler or in toaster oven or microwave until cheese melts and bubbles.

Yield: 8 pizzas

Nutritive values per 1-pizza serving:	CAL	CHO (gm)	PRO (gm)	FAT (gm)
	218	18	13	11

Food exchanges per 1-pizza serving: 1 BREAD, 1½ medium-fat MEAT, ½ VEGETABLE

Sloppy Joes

1 pound lean ground beef
½ onion, chopped fine
2 stalks celery, including leaves, chopped
½ green pepper, chopped
2 medium fresh tomatoes, pureed in blender
2 tablespoons fresh lemon juice
½ teaspoon dry mustard
2 teaspoons Worcestershire sauce
3 whole wheat hamburger buns, split and
toasted

1. Put meat in heavy frying pan and cook over medium heat until brown. Drain in a colander to rid of all fat.
2. Combine remaining ingredients, except hamburger buns, in pan and sauté over medium heat for 5 minutes. Add meat, reduce heat, and simmer, covered, for 15 minutes more. Stir frequently.
3. Serve on hamburger bun half.

Yield: 6 servings

Nutritive values per serving (including ½ cup meat mixture):	CAL	CHO (gm)	PRO (gm)	FAT (gm)
	196	18	17	6

Food exchanges per serving
(including ½ cup meat mixture): 1 BREAD, 2 lean MEAT,
1 VEGETABLE

MAIN COURSE LUNCHES
Baked Macaroni and Cheese

   1 cup whole wheat or regular elbow macaroni
   2 eggs, beaten
   1 cup skim milk
   1 cup low-fat cottage cheese
  ¼ cup shredded extra-sharp Cheddar cheese
  ½ teaspoon dry mustard
  ¼ teaspoon ground white pepper
   1 tablespoon dry bread crumbs

1. Preheat oven to 350°F.
2. Cook macaroni according to package instructions, without salt. Drain.
3. Combine macaroni with next 6 ingredients. Spoon into a 1-quart baking dish that has been wiped with a little bit of oil. Sprinkle with bread crumbs. Bake for 1 hour.

Yield: 6 ⅔-cup servings

Nutritive values per ⅔-cup serving:	CAL	CHO (gm)	PRO (gm)	FAT (gm)
	179	17	12	7

Food exchanges per ⅔-cup serving:

1 BREAD, 1½ medium-fat MEAT

Baked Beans

1 pound dried northern beans
Cold water
½ cup chopped center-cut ham (bone, fat, and
   skin removed)
1 cup chopped onions
1 6-ounce can tomato paste
1 teaspoon salt
2 tablespoons Dijon mustard
1 tablespoon vinegar
2 tablespoons blackstrap molasses
8 packets artificial sweetener (equal to ⅓ cup
   sugar)

1. Wash and sort beans. Add cold water, cover, and soak
   overnight.
2. The next day, drain and cover with fresh cold water.
   Bring to boil and simmer for 30 minutes. Preheat oven
   to 250°F.
3. Drain and reserve bean liquid. Mix beans with remaining ingredients and place in a covered baking dish.
4. Bake for 6–9 hours in oven or use crock pot on low
   setting. Add reserved bean water if they become dry.
   Uncover for the last hour of cooking.

Yield: 6 cups (18 servings)

Nutritive values per ⅓-cup serving:	CAL	CHO (gm)	PRO (gm)	FAT (gm)
	126	19	8	2

Food exchanges per ⅓-cup
serving: 1 BREAD, ½ lean MEAT, 1
                                 VEGETABLE

Turkey Chili

This is an easy, very tasty dish, and turkey is much lower in fat than beef or pork. You can use strips of leftover roast turkey instead of uncooked ground turkey, about 4 cups, and add it to the beans for the last 10 minutes of cooking time. To use dried beans, cover 1 cup of beans with water and simmer for 1 hour or until tender; they will yield 2 cups cooked.

2 pounds ground turkey
1 medium onion, chopped
2 cloves garlic, pressed or minced
1 16-ounce can whole tomatoes, undrained
1 8-ounce can tomato sauce
2 cups homemade chicken stock
1 fresh Anaheim chili, seeded and chopped (optional)
2 tablespoons chili powder or more to taste
1 teaspoon ground cumin
1 teaspoon paprika
½ teaspoon freshly ground pepper
2 green apples, peeled and chopped
2 cups cooked red or pinto beans *or* 1 16-ounce can, drained

1. Combine all ingredients except apples and beans in large pot. Bring to a boil, reduce heat, cover, and simmer for 30 minutes. Stir frequently to break up the turkey and tomatoes.
2. Add apples and simmer covered for another 20 minutes. Add beans and cook 10 minutes longer.

Yield: 8 1⅓-cup servings

Nutritive values per 1⅓-cup serving:	CAL	CHO (gm)	PRO (gm)	FAT (gm)
	261	20	25	0

Food exchanges per 1⅓-cup serving:

1 BREAD, 3 lean MEAT, 1 VEGETABLE

Chili Deluxe with Vegetables

These are sneaky vegetables, the kind your kids hardly notice. They add nutrition and fiber while playing second fiddle to the meat and beans.

1 cup dried pinto beans
1 pound lean ground beef
1 large onion, chopped
2 cloves garlic, pressed or minced
2 tablespoons chili powder
1 teaspoon paprika
¼ teaspoon ground cloves
½ teaspoon ground cumin
½ teaspoon ground coriander
½ teaspoon oregano leaves
½ teaspoon basil leaves
1 8-ounce can tomato sauce
1 16-ounce can tomatoes
1 cup homemade beef or chicken stock
1 cup diced green pepper
1 cup grated carrots
1 cup diced celery

1. Cook beans in water to cover for 1 hour or until just tender. Drain and set aside.
2. Sauté beef, onion, and garlic for 10 minutes. Drain off all fat.
3. Add seasonings, tomato sauce, tomatoes, and stock and simmer for 1 hour. Add more stock if necessary.
4. Add green pepper, carrots, and celery and cook, covered, for 20 minutes, until tender. Add beans and heat for 10 minutes.

Yield: 8 1-cup servings

Nutritive values per 1-cup serving:	CAL	CHO (gm)	PRO (gm)	FAT (gm)
	219	25	19	5

Food exchanges per 1-cup serving:

1 BREAD, 2 lean MEAT, 2 VEGETABLE

SALADS
New Potato Salad

2 pounds small red new potatoes
½ small red onion, chopped
1 green pepper, seeded and chopped
2 hard-cooked eggs, chopped
¼ cup minced fresh parsley
1 cup plain nonfat yogurt
2 tablespoons diet mayonnaise
3 tablespoons minced fresh dill *or* 1
   tablespoon dried dill weed
2 tablespoons Dijon mustard
1 tablespoon fresh lemon juice
½ teaspoon freshly ground pepper
   Paprika

1. Steam the potatoes, unpeeled, until they are just tender when pierced with a fork. If small, halve them. If medium-size, quarter them. Use a sharp knife and try not to pull the skin off.
2. Add the onion, green pepper, eggs, and parsley.
3. Combine yogurt, mayonnaise, dill, mustard, lemon juice, and pepper and pour over vegetables. Mix gently. Sprinkle with paprika and refrigerate.

Yield: 8 ⅔-cup servings

Nutritive values per ⅔-cup serving:	CAL	CHO (gm)	PRO (gm)	FAT (gm)
	149	21	5	5

Food exchanges per ⅔-cup serving: 1½ BREAD, 1 FAT

German Potato Salad

This is an Italian version of German potato salad because it uses pancetta instead of bacon. Pancetta is a bacon-type meat that is preserved with salt, not nitrates, and can be found in Italian delis. You can use bacon if you absolutely have to, but try to get pancetta.

4 medium potatoes, peeled
1 medium onion, chopped
3 stalks celery, chopped
2 teaspoons olive oil
½ cup water
6 tablespoons cider vinegar
1 tablespoon all-purpose flour
2 packets artificial sweetener (equal to 4 teaspoons sugar)
½ teaspoon freshly ground pepper
2 tablespoons minced fresh parsley
2 ounces pancetta, chopped, sautéed until crisp, and drained

1. Cook potatoes in boiling water to cover until tender, about 25–30 minutes. Drain.
2. Fry onion and celery in olive oil until onion is slightly browned. Add water, vinegar, flour, sweetener, and pepper. Cook and stir over medium heat until thickened, about 10 minutes.
3. Slice potatoes and place in bowl. Add parsley and pancetta. Pour sauce over and mix gently.

Yield: 4 cups (8 servings)

Nutritive values per ½-cup serving:	CAL	CHO (gm)	PRO (gm)	FAT (gm)
	108	20	4	3

Food exchanges per ½-cup serving: 1 BREAD, 1 VEGETABLE, ½ FAT

Coleslaw

4 cups shredded green cabbage
2 cups shredded carrots
¾ cup thinly sliced green onions
⅔ cup cider vinegar
1 tablespoon Dijon mustard
1½ teaspoons paprika
1 teaspoon mustard seeds
½ teaspoon celery seeds
½ teaspoon freshly ground pepper
½ cup nonfat yogurt
½ cup low-fat cottage cheese

1. Combine cabbage, carrots, and onions in a large bowl.
2. Combine remaining ingredients in a blender or food processor and whirl just until smooth. Pour over vegetables and refrigerate overnight.

Yield: 8 1-cup servings

Nutritive values per 1-cup serving:	CAL	CHO (gm)	PRO (gm)	FAT (gm)
	49	6	4	1

Food exchanges per 1-cup serving: 1 VEGETABLE, trace FAT

Special Fruited Coleslaw

1 small green cabbage (approximately 1½ pounds), chopped
1 20-ounce can unsweetened crushed pineapple, undrained
2 medium apples, diced
1½ cups grated carrots
1 cup chopped celery
½ cup golden raisins
1 cup nonfat yogurt
1 teaspoon grated lemon zest
1 teaspoon fresh lemon juice

Combine all ingredients in a large bowl and toss. Cover and refrigerate overnight.

Yield: 11 1-cup servings

Nutritive values per 1-cup serving:	CAL	CHO (gm)	PRO (gm)	FAT (gm)
	90	20	3	0

Food exchanges per 1-cup serving: 1 FRUIT, 2 VEGETABLE

8
Snacks

Snack time can be easy or frustrating, depending on your child's tastes and flexibility. If her snack exchanges are a BREAD and a FRUIT, it's easy to put 10 Wheat Thins and an apple in front of her. Your child, however, may not feel like eating Wheat Thins and an apple. That's why many recipes in this chapter combine BREAD and FRUIT or BREAD and MEAT exchanges in the form of nutritious, special snacks and treats.

No two days are exactly alike for a child. It is always best to stick as closely as possible to your child's prescribed diet plan, but, as parents, we learn things about our children's reactions to different foods that no doctor or dietitian can predict in advance. For a long time, Brennan has had very different day-to-day afternoon blood sugars, so a set amount of food in the afternoon is not a good idea in Brennan's case. This is why blood-testing has become so important to us, as it should be for your child. Brennan may come home really hungry and yet have a 180 blood sugar. Then I try to fill him up with vegetables and dip and a noncaloric drink. Other days, he's 130 but has soccer or basketball practice. That's a good time for an extra treat like frozen yogurt or ice cream.

Concerning frozen desserts, many of the yogurt and even ice cream parlors now make a very healthy version that is low-fat, sweetened with fructose, and uses unsweetened berries for toppings. An interesting note on ice cream and such is that, of all the parents I talked to, none mentioned that ice cream raised their child's blood sugar unreasonably. Quite the opposite, in fact: several said ice cream was fine but other foods, like pizza, sent blood sugars through the roof. I asked Tina Leeser, the nutritionist for this book, why. She hypothesized that many of the less expensive ice creams are made with guar, which is a gel-like fiber that holds the food in the stomach longer. That way, the food takes longer to metabolize and raises the blood sugar more slowly. Nutrition researcher Phyllis Crapo noted that even ice creams made without guar rated lower than many foods on the glycemic index. Researchers aren't sure why.

Snack time is time to think of good nutrition, not just feeding your child anything that's a bread or a fruit exchange. The closer to a natural state a food is, the better. Whole grain bread is far better than crackers, whole fruit is better than juice, etc. The usual good sense should prevail. All the snacks in this chapter are good sources of nutrition.

This chapter is divided into three sections: beverages, savory snacks, and sweet snacks. Generally, you'll find the quickest recipes to prepare in the earlier pages of this chapter. Shakes are a snap to prepare, and the savory snacks resemble simple appetizers.

Diet sodas present a bit of a dilemma at our house. I would prefer that my boys not drink sodas—diet or otherwise. They add nothing to their overall health. They often contain added chemicals and sodium, and phosphates, which can interfere with absorption of calcium when ingested in large amounts. Instead of banning them, I encourage moderation. I try to limit our consumption of diet sodas as much as possible, so we use flavored mineral water and Crystal Light for noncaloric drinks. There are now several sugar-free, noncarbonated drink mixes on the market. (The healthiest beverage, of course, is water, but I know my kids want something flavored most of the time.)

Many of the recipes in the sweet snacks section would normally pass as desserts. They are listed in this chapter, rather than as dinner recipes, because I would rather serve a treat-type snack in the morning or afternoon when a child is active.

SNACK EXCHANGES

Use this list as a quick reference when planning snack menus. A glance at the right-hand column should give you ideas of what to serve for certain exchanges called for in your child's diet plan. The recipes are listed here in the same order as they appear in the chapter.

Pineapple Shake	1 FRUIT, ½ MILK
Chocolate Shake	1 MILK
Grape Soda	1 FRUIT
Spiced Tea	Less than 1 cup FREE; 1 cup = ½ FRUIT
Dip for Vegetables or Sort-of Sour Cream	1 lean MEAT
Bean Dip	1⅓ BREAD
Peanut Dip	1 FAT
Homemade Tortilla Chips	1 BREAD, ½ FAT
Sesame Nachos	½ BREAD, 1 FAT
Popcorn Treat	1½ BREAD, ½ FRUIT, ½ FAT
Meatball Snacks	1 lean MEAT
Devilish Eggs	½ medium-fat MEAT
Peach Whip	½ FRUIT
Frozen Banana	½ BREAD, 1 FRUIT
Frozen Fruit Pops	⅔ FRUIT
Orange Sherbert	1 FRUIT, ½ MILK
Pineapple Sherbert	1½ FRUIT
Carrot and Raisin Salad	½ FRUIT, 1 VEGETABLE, trace FAT
Apple Salad	1 FRUIT, trace FAT
Baked Custard	½ MILK, ½ lean MEAT
Brennan's Rice Pudding	1 BREAD, ½ lean MEAT, ½ FAT
Peanut Butter Cookies	1 BREAD, ½ FRUIT, 2 FAT
Chocolate Chip Cookies	1 BREAD, 1½ FAT
"Wholesome" Brownies	1 FRUIT, 1½ FAT

Apple Crunch	1 BREAD, 1 FRUIT, 1 FAT
Oatmeal Cookies	½ BREAD, ½ FAT
Cherry Pie	⅔ BREAD, 1 FRUIT, 1 FAT
Lean Pie Crust	½ BREAD, ½ FAT
Quick Banana Cream Pie	1 BREAD, ½ FRUIT, ½ MILK, 1 FAT
Graham Cracker Crust	1 BREAD, 1 FAT
Fresh Peach Pie	1 BREAD, 1½ FRUIT, 1 FAT
Whole Grain Pastry Shell	1 BREAD, 1 FAT
Applesauce Bran Squares	1 BREAD, 1½ FAT
Carrot Snack Cake	1 BREAD, ½ FRUIT, 1 FAT
Vanilla Cheesecake	½ BREAD, 1 MILK, 2 FAT
Oatmeal Bread	1 BREAD, ½ FRUIT, ½ FAT
Zucchini Bread	⅔ BREAD, 1 FAT

Recipes

BEVERAGES

Pineapple Shake

A child any age can help you make this shake. Toddlers can count out the pineapple pieces and help measure the flavoring. Older children can whip it up themselves.

½ cup skim milk
10 pieces unsweetened canned pineapple
     chunks and small amount of juice
     (approximately ½ cup)
1 packet artificial sweetener (Equal)
1 teaspoon pineapple flavoring
1 teaspoon coconut flavoring

Blend all ingredients in blender or food processor. Blend until smooth.

Yield: 1 serving

Nutritive values per serving:	CAL	CHO (gm)	PRO (gm)	FAT (gm)
	80	16	4	0

Food exchanges per serving: 1 FRUIT, ½ MILK

Chocolate Shake

Commercial sugar-free chocolate milk mixes are now available, or you can make this one. Better yet, teach your child to make it!

>   1 cup skim milk
>   1 tablespoon unsweetened cocoa
>   1 packet artificial sweetener (Equal)
>   3–4 ice cubes

Place ingredients in blender or food processor and blend at high speed until frothy and thickened. Serve immediately.

Yield: 1 serving

Nutritive values per serving:

CAL	CHO (gm)	PRO (gm)	FAT (gm)
100	15	9	0

Food exchanges per serving: 1 MILK

Grape Soda

>   ¼ cup unsweetened grape juice
>   1 cup sparkling water

Variations

1. To make apple soda, replace ingredients above with ⅓ cup unsweetened apple juice and 1 cup lemon-lime-flavored diet soda.
2. To make orange soda, use ½ cup unsweetened orange juice and 1 cup lemon-lime-flavored diet soda.

Yield: 1 serving

Nutritive values per serving:

CAL	CHO (gm)	PRO (gm)	FAT (gm)
40	10	0	0

Food exchanges per serving: 1 FRUIT

Spiced Tea

I first had this in Canada and thought it was a very refreshing drink, hot or iced. This version uses herb tea since children certainly don't need caffeine.

> 6 cups boiling water
> 8 whole cloves
> 3 cinnamon sticks
> 6 bags herb orange/spice tea (noncaffeinated)
> 1 6-ounce can unsweetened pineapple juice
> 1 cup unsweetened orange juice
> Juice of ½ lemon
> 4 packets artificial sweetener (Equal)

Simmer the water and spices for 5 minutes. Add tea bags and remove from heat. Steep for 5 minutes. Remove tea bags and spices. Add juices and sweetener. Serve immediately or refrigerate in covered pitcher. Reheat or serve iced.

Yield: 8 1-cup servings

Nutritive values per 1-cup serving:	CAL	CHO (gm)	PRO (gm)	FAT (gm)
	16	4	0	0

Food exchanges per 1-cup serving: Less than 1 cup FREE; 1 cup = ½ FRUIT

SAVORY SNACKS

Dip for Vegetables, or Sort-of Sour Cream

Use this recipe as a base for dips or as a replacement for sour cream on baked potatoes. My kids don't notice any difference between this and the higher-fat sour cream dips. Brennan loves to add the herbs and spices. A dip like this is great after school, surrounded by whatever vegetables your child likes. Be inventive and try Chinese pea pods, fresh green beans, jicama strips, green or red pepper strips, broccoli and cauliflower flowerets, as well as the old standbys of carrots, celery, and cucumber. Your child may develop a liking for a new vegetable if it's served with a tasty dip.

½ cup plain nonfat yogurt
½ cup low-fat cottage cheese
1 tablespoon fresh lemon juice or white vinegar

Combine the ingredients in a blender or food processor and blend briefly, until smooth. Chill an hour or two, after adding whatever herbs and spices you desire, or use the following variations.

Variations
1. Add 2 tablespoons chopped fresh parsley, 1 clove finely minced garlic, and dash cayenne pepper to dip mixture before chilling.
2. Add 2 tablespoons chopped fresh dill, chives, cilantro, basil, or tarragon (*or* 2 teaspoons dried) or a combination of these herbs to dip mixture before chilling.
3. Add 2 tablespoons Parmesan cheese and 2 tablespoons chopped fresh chives to dip mixture before chilling.

Yield: 1 cup

Nutritive values per 3-tablespoon serving:	CAL	CHO (gm)	PRO (gm)	FAT (gm)
	43	1	7	trace

Food exchanges per 3-tablespoon serving: 1 lean MEAT

Bean Dip

Serve this dip with Tortilla Chips (recipe follows). You can buy canned bean dip, but making your own is easy. It's also healthier because it will be much lower in sodium. Legumes raise the blood sugar slowly, so they are good for diabetics.

> 2 cups cooked pinto beans *or* 1 16-ounce can pinto beans
> 2 tablespoons finely chopped canned or fresh green chilies, seeded, *or* 1 fresh jalapeño, seeded and minced (optional)
> 1 tablespoon fresh lemon juice
> 1 tablespoon red wine vinegar
> 1 teaspoon chili powder
> 1 teaspoon ground cumin
> 1 tablespoon minced fresh cilantro or parsley

Place all ingredients in a blender or food processor and blend until smooth. Serve at room temperature.

Yield: 2 cups

Nutritive values per 2-tablespoon serving:	CAL	CHO (gm)	PRO (gm)	FAT (gm)
	42	22	2	trace

Food exchanges per 2-tablespoon serving: 1⅓ BREAD

Peanut Dip

The first time I tried this recipe I thought it would be either awful or wonderful. It's wonderful! Serve it with celery sticks, cucumber slices, jicama strips, and/or fresh pineapple chunks. (You can use canned pineapple, but fresh is much better.) Peanut butter is a concentrated source of calories, but, according to our knowledge of glycemic reaction, the fat content should assist in slowing the rise of blood sugar. The fiber in the fresh vegetables and fruit will also help to slow blood sugar rise. Remember also that peanut oil is a monounsaturated fat and may actually help cholesterol problems. For those reasons, an extra serving shouldn't be a problem for an active child. I say all of this because 2 tablespoons might look like a paltry serving. Put it in the center of a small plate and surround it with raw vegetables and ½ cup pineapple chunks (1 FRUIT). It's a filling snack.

⅓ cup smooth or crunchy natural peanut butter
2 packets artificial sweetener (Equal)
¼ cup fresh lemon juice
2 tablespoons tomato-based chili sauce or catsup
½ teaspoon soy sauce
Dash cayenne pepper

Mix all ingredients together and serve at room temperature.

Yield: ⅔ cup

Nutritive values per 2-tablespoon serving:		CHO	PRO	FAT
	CAL	(gm)	(gm)	(gm)
	52	2	2	4

Food exchanges per 2-tablespoon serving: 1 FAT

Homemade Tortilla Chips

*These chips are superior to commercial chips for two
healthy reasons—lower sodium and much lower fat.*

> 10 6-inch fresh corn tortillas
> 2 tablespoons peanut or vegetable oil

1. Preheat oven to 350°F.
2. Using a pastry brush, lightly coat one side of each
tortilla with oil. Use a sharp knife to cut the tortillas,
stacked together, into halves, quarters, then eighths.
3. Spread chips on nonstick baking pans. Bake for 10
minutes or until crisp and beginning to brown.

Yield: 80 chips

Nutritive values per 10-chip serving:	CAL	CHO (gm)	PRO (gm)	FAT (gm)
	90	15	2	2

Food exchanges per 10-chip
serving: 1 BREAD, ½ FAT

Sesame Nachos

*Everybody loves these, and kids can easily make them
on their own.*

> 4 Homemade Tortilla Chips (see previous
>   recipe)
> 4 tablespoons grated Cheddar cheese
> 1 tablespoon unhulled sesame seeds

Top the chips with cheese and sesame seeds. Broil just
until cheese melts, or use your toaster oven or microwave
on medium for 1½–2½ minutes, just until cheese melts.

Yield: 1 serving

Nutritive values per serving:	CAL	CHO (gm)	PRO (gm)	FAT (gm)
	82	4	3	6

Food exchanges per serving: ½ BREAD, 1 FAT

Popcorn Treat

This is a good, healthy after-school snack that can be made in larger quantities and stored in an airtight container at room temperature.

    1 cup plain popped popcorn (unsalted, preferably air-popped)
    1 cup bite-size shredded wheat biscuits
    2 tablespoons raisins
    1 tablespoon dry-roasted sunflower seeds
  ½ teaspoon ground cinnamon

Mix first 4 ingredients. Sprinkle cinnamon over mixture and toss lightly.

Yield: 2 cups (2 servings)

Nutritive values per 1-cup serving:	CAL	CHO (gm)	PRO (gm)	FAT (gm)
	150	27	3	3

Food exchanges per 1-cup serving:

1½ BREAD, ½ FRUIT, ½ FAT

Meatball Snacks

This is a variation of a recipe from The Art of Cooking for the Diabetic, *by Katharine Middleton and Mary Abbott Hess (Contemporary Books, 1978).*

    1 pound very lean ground beef
    1 large egg, beaten
  ¼ cup tomato juice
  ¼ teaspoon ground nutmeg
    1 teaspoon grated lemon zest
    2 tablespoons fresh lemon juice
    2 tablespoons wheat germ
    1 slice fresh whole grain bread, finely crumbled

1. Preheat oven to 400°F.
2. Line a shallow baking pan with foil or use a nonstick pan.
3. Combine all ingredients and mix well. Form into tiny balls, using about 1 teaspoon of mixture per ball. Place 1 inch apart in pan. Bake 10 minutes.

Yield: 80 meatballs (20 servings)

Nutritive values per 4-meatball serving:	CAL	CHO (gm)	PRO (gm)	FAT (gm)
	51	1	5	3

Food exchanges per 4-meatball serving: 1 lean MEAT

Devilish Eggs

This is a good high-protein snack to serve occasionally with vegetables and dip. I recommend serving it only occasionally because the egg yolks are high in cholesterol.

8 hard-cooked eggs
½ cup low-fat cottage cheese
1 tablespoon Dijon mustard
   Dash hot red pepper sauce

1. Cut eggs in half lengthwise. Remove yolks.
2. Mash yolks with remaining ingredients and spoon mixture back into egg whites.

Yield: 16 stuffed halves (8 servings)

Nutritive values per 1-piece serving:	CAL	CHO (gm)	PRO (gm)	FAT (gm)
	39	0	4	3

Food exchanges per 1-piece serving: ½ medium-fat MEAT

SWEET SNACKS

Peach Whip

This recipe is from General Foods, the maker of Jell-O.

- ¾ cup boiling water
- 1 4-serving package sugar-free orange or raspberry Jell-O
- ½ cup ice cubes
- 1 8-ounce can sliced peaches in juice or light syrup

1. Pour water into blender or food processor with gelatin. Blend until dissolved. Add ice cubes and stir until partially melted.

2. Drain peaches. Add to gelatin and blend until ice is melted and peaches are pureed. Pour into serving bowl or glasses. Chill about 2 hours, until set.

Yield: 4 servings (approximately 2 cups)

Nutritive values per ½-cup serving:	CAL	CHO (gm)	PRO (gm)	FAT (gm)
	24	5	1	0

Food exchanges per ½-cup serving: ½ FRUIT

Frozen Banana

My kids love the frozen bananas we buy at amusement parks. Those are usually coated with chocolate, but these are good, too. Make several and have them ready for a snack.

$\frac{1}{2}$ banana, peeled
2 tablespoons skim milk
$\frac{1}{4}$ cup Grape Nuts cereal, crushed to crumbs
    Dash each ground cinnamon and ground
    nutmeg

1. Insert an ice cream stick deeply into the cut end of the banana.
2. Dip the banana in milk and roll in cereal crumbs and spices.
3. Wrap in plastic and freeze.

Yield: 1 serving

Nutritive values per serving:	CAL	CHO (gm)	PRO (gm)	FAT (gm)
	68	16	1	0

Food exchanges per serving: $\frac{1}{2}$ BREAD, 1 FRUIT

Frozen Fruit Pops

Like most kids, mine love Popsicles, especially in the summer. These frozen fruit pops are so much better for your child than anything you can buy. They contain no added sugar and have the added benefit of fiber from the banana. Tupperware makes good frozen bar forms that I use all the time. Use the following recipe or ¼ cup unsweetened grape or orange juice in each form, which would equal 1 FRUIT. The exchanges below are based on ¼ cup per frozen fruit pop; ⅓ cup would be almost 1 FRUIT.

>   1 cup mashed ripe banana
>   1 8-ounce can unsweetened crushed
>   pineapple, undrained
>   1 cup unsweetened orange juice
>   2 teaspoons fresh lemon juice

1. Combine all ingredients and pour into 8- or 9-inch baking pan. Freeze until almost firm.
2. Spoon mixture into a mixing bowl and beat with an electric mixer until smooth and creamy. Spoon mixture into frozen bar forms. Freeze until firm.

Yield: 12 frozen fruit treats

Nutritive values per frozen fruit pop:	CAL	CHO (gm)	PRO (gm)	FAT (gm)
	28	7	0	0

Food exchanges per frozen fruit pop: ⅔ FRUIT

Orange Sherbert

>   1 6-ounce can orange juice concentrate
>   1½ cups skim milk
>   ⅔ cup nonfat dry milk
>   1 teaspoon vanilla extract

1. Blend ingredients well and put in freezer until partially frozen—45 minutes to 1 hour.
2. Remove from freezer and beat until smooth. Return to
freezer until frozen.

Yield: 6 ½-cup servings

Nutritive values per ½-cup serving:	CAL	CHO (gm)	PRO (gm)	FAT (gm)
	88	18	4	0

Food exchanges per ½-cup
serving: 1 FRUIT, ½ MILK

Pineapple Sherbert

8 ounces nonfat yogurt
1 20-ounce can unsweetened crushed
   pineapple in juice
4 packets artificial sweetener (Equal)
½ cup unsweetened orange juice

1. Combine all ingredients in blender or food processor.
Whirl 1 minute, pour into shallow baking pan, and
freeze until frozen 1 inch around edges.
2. Turn into chilled bowl and beat with electric or rotary
beater until smooth, then freeze until set.
3. Allow to soften slightly at room temperature before
serving.

Yield: 8 ½-cup servings

Nutritive values per ½-cup serving:	CAL	CHO (gm)	PRO (gm)	FAT (gm)
	73	16	1	0

Food exchanges per ½-cup
serving: 1½ FRUIT

Carrot and Raisin Salad

Some kids love this sort of dish, and some don't, but it's so nutritious that it's worth a try.

    4 medium carrots, grated
    ½ cup golden raisins
    ¼ cup nonfat yogurt
    ¼ cup low-fat cottage cheese
    1½ teaspoons fresh lemon juice
    1 packet artificial sweetener (Equal)
    ⅛ teaspoon cayenne pepper (optional)

1. Combine carrots and raisins.
2. Combine remaining ingredients in blender or food processor. Whirl until smooth. Stir into carrot mixture.

Yield: 6 ½-cup servings

Nutritive values per ½-cup serving:	CAL	CHO (gm)	PRO (gm)	FAT (gm)
	47	7	3	1

Food exchanges per ½-cup serving:

½ FRUIT, 1 VEGETABLE, trace FAT

Apple Salad

This easy and delicious salad is from Jane Brody's Good Food Book.

Salad
2 large red delicious apples, cored but unpeeled and cut into chunks
⅔ cup canned crushed unsweetened pineapple, drained, or fresh minced pineapple, juice reserved
⅓ cup diced celery
2 tablespoons raisins

Dressing
3 tablespoons low-fat yogurt
2 teaspoons diet mayonnaise
1 tablespoon pineapple juice (reserved from pineapple)
⅛ teaspoon ground cinnamon

1. In a medium bowl, combine the salad ingredients.
2. In a small bowl, combine the dressing ingredients. Add the dressing to the fruit mixture and blend.

Yield: 8 ½-cup servings

Nutritive values per ½-cup serving:	CAL	CHO (gm)	PRO (gm)	FAT (gm)
	41	8	0	1

Food exchanges per ½-cup serving: 1 FRUIT, trace FAT

Baked Custard

1   12-ounce can evaporated skim milk
2   eggs, beaten slightly
1   egg white
2   tablespoons sugar
4   packets artificial sweetener (equal to 8
    teaspoons sugar)
1   teaspoon vanilla extract
½   teaspoon grated orange or lemon zest
¼   teaspoon ground nutmeg or mace

1. Preheat oven to 325°F.
2. Heat milk in the top of a double boiler over simmering water until surface begins to wrinkle.
3. Blend together the eggs, egg white, sugar, sweetener, vanilla, and zest. Add hot milk gradually, stirring to mix well.
4. Pour into 4 individual custard cups. Sprinkle with nutmeg. Set cups in a pan; pour hot water around cups to within ½ inch of tops of custard cups. Bake 50–60 minutes or until knife tip inserted in center of custard comes out clean. Chill several hours before serving.

Yield: 4 ½-cup servings

Nutritive values per ½-cup serving:	CAL	CHO (gm)	PRO (gm)	FAT (gm)
	87	6	9	3

Food exchanges per ½-cup
serving: ½ MILK, ½ lean MEAT

Brennan's Rice Pudding

3 eggs
6 packets artificial sweetener (equal to ¼ cup
  sugar)
2 teaspoons vanilla extract
¼ teaspoon each ground cinnamon and
  ground nutmeg
2 cups evaporated skim milk
1 cup long-grain brown rice or white
  converted rice, cooked
¼ cup raisins

1. Preheat oven to 325°F.
2. Beat eggs. Mix in sweetener, vanilla, cinnamon, and
nutmeg.
3. Add milk and mix thoroughly. Stir in rice and raisins.
Pour into 2-quart soufflé dish. Place in shallow pan
and pour hot water around soufflé dish to a depth of
1 inch. Bake for approximately 45 minutes.

Yield: 8 ½-cup servings

Nutritive values per ½-cup serving:	CAL	CHO (gm)	PRO (gm)	FAT (gm)
	113	15	9	2

Food exchanges per ½-cup
serving: 1 BREAD, ½ lean MEAT, ½ FAT

Peanut Butter Cookies

These cookies contain only ½ teaspoon of sugar per cookie, and my boys love them.

1½ cups sifted unbleached white flour
1½ teaspoons double-acting baking powder
½ teaspoon salt
¼ cup diet margarine
¼ cup brown sugar or fructose
½ cup smooth, natural peanut butter (no added sugar or hydrogenated oils)
1 teaspoon grated fresh orange zest
2 teaspoons vanilla extract
1 egg, well beaten
⅓ cup unsweetened orange juice
4 packets artificial sweetener (equal to 8 teaspoons sugar)

1. Preheat oven to 400°F.
2. Sift together flour, baking powder, and salt.
3. Cream together margarine, sugar, peanut butter, orange zest, and vanilla. Add egg, orange juice, and sweetener; blend well.
4. Add dry ingredients gradually; mix well after each addition.
5. Measure 1 level tablespoon dough for each cookie. Roll between hands to form ball. Place 2 inches apart on an ungreased cookie sheet; flatten with fork. Bake about 15 minutes. Store cookies in a tightly covered tin. These cookies have better flavor and texture 24 hours after baking.

Yield: 24 cookies

Nutritive values per 2-cookie serving:	CAL	CHO (gm)	PRO (gm)	FAT (gm)
	170	17	5	9

Food exchanges per 2-cookie serving: 1 BREAD, ½ FRUIT, 2 FAT

Chocolate Chip Cookies

This recipe comes from The New Diabetic Cookbook, *by Mabel Cavaiani (Contemporary Books, 1984).*

1 cup (2 sticks) diet margarine at room temperature
¼ cup sugar
¼ cup Brown SugarTwin
3 large egg whites at room temperature
1 tablespoon vanilla extract
2 cups unbleached white flour
1 teaspoon baking soda
¼ teaspoon salt
¼ cup water at room temperature
½ cup mini semisweet chocolate chips

1. Preheat oven to 375°F.
2. Cream margarine, sugar, and Brown SugarTwin at medium speed until light and fluffy. Add egg whites and vanilla to creamed mixture and beat at medium speed for 1 minute.
3. Stir together flour, soda, and salt to blend well. Add water to creamed mixture along with the flour mixture and mix at medium speed for 1 minute or until smooth.
4. Add chocolate chips to dough and mix lightly. Drop by tablespoonfuls onto cookie sheets that have been lined with aluminum foil or are nonstick. Press down lightly with fingers dipped in cold water to form a circle about 2 inches across. Bake about 12–15 minutes or until browned. (The cookies won't be crisp unless they are browned.)

Yield: 44 cookies

Nutritive values per 2-cookie serving:	CAL	CHO (gm)	PRO (gm)	FAT (gm)
	144	15	3	8

Food exchanges per 2-cookie serving: 1 BREAD, 1½ FAT

"Wholesome" Brownies

These delicious brownies are courtesy of Jane Brody's Good Food Book. *The oats and wheat germ add nutrition and high fiber, which slows down the rise of blood sugar. The sugar content is about 1 teaspoon per brownie. If you have any concern about the sugar content, please consult your dietitian or physician.*

> 1   6-ounce package (1 cup) semisweet chocolate chips
> ⅓   cup diet margarine
> 1   scant cup quick-cooking rolled oats
> ¼   cup wheat germ
> ⅓   cup nonfat dry milk
> ½   teaspoon double-acting baking powder
> ¼   teaspoon salt (optional)
> ½   cup chopped walnuts
> 2   eggs
> ¼   cup packed brown sugar
> 2   tablespoons white sugar
> 1   teaspoon vanilla extract

1. Preheat oven to 350°F.
2. In the top of a double boiler or in a small heavy saucepan over very low heat, melt the chocolate chips and the margarine. Remove the pan from the heat and stir the mixture until it is smooth. Set it aside.
3. In a medium bowl, combine the oats, wheat germ, dry milk, baking powder, salt, and nuts. Set the mixture aside.
4. In a large mixing bowl, beat the eggs and mix in the brown and white sugars and the vanilla until the mixture is thick. Stir in the melted chocolate mixture. Fold in the oats mixture until it is just blended. Pour the batter into a greased 8-inch square baking pan.
5. Bake the brownies for 20–25 minutes or until the top is crisp but a toothpick inserted in the center of the pan comes out slightly moist. Set pan on a rack to cool completely before cutting the brownies into 5 strips in each direction.

Yield: 25 brownies

Nutritive values per 1-brownie serving:	CAL	CHO (gm)	PRO (gm)	FAT (gm)
	111	10	2	7

Food exchanges per 1-brownie serving: 1 FRUIT, 1½ FAT

Apple Crunch

This is a good alternative to apple pie and one my kids love. Lemon juice can be used instead of lime, but lime is more interesting.

    4 cups pared, sliced apples
    ¾ cup unsweetened orange juice
    1 teaspoon fresh lime juice
    1 teaspoon ground cinnamon
    1 cup graham cracker crumbs
    2 tablespoons wheat germ
    2 tablespoons diet margarine

1. Preheat oven to 400°F.
2. Layer apples in 1-quart casserole. Combine juices and cinnamon and pour over apples.
3. Combine cracker crumbs and wheat germ with margarine and sprinkle over apples.
4. Cover with foil and bake for 25 minutes. Uncover and bake 5–10 minutes longer.

Yield: 10 ⅓-cup servings

Nutritive values per ⅓-cup serving:	CAL	CHO (gm)	PRO (gm)	FAT (gm)
	153	25	2	5

Food exchanges per ⅓-cup serving: 1 BREAD, 1 FRUIT, 1 FAT

Oatmeal Cookies

These cookies are a good snack because the oatmeal provides protein and fiber to raise blood sugar slowly.

⅓ cup raisins
¾ cup boiling water
¼ cup brown sugar
6 packets artificial sweetener (equal to ¼ cup sugar)
1 cup (2 sticks) diet margarine at room temperature
1 egg
2 egg whites
1 teaspoon vanilla extract
2 cups unbleached white flour
1½ teaspoons ground cinnamon
1 teaspoon double-acting baking powder
½ teaspoon baking soda
2 cups rolled oats (regular or quick, not instant)

1. Preheat oven to 375°F.
2. Combine raisins and boiling water and set aside to cool to room temperature.
3. Cream together sugar, sweetener, and margarine at medium speed until light and fluffy. Add egg, egg whites, and vanilla to creamed mixture and mix at low speed for 1 minute.
4. Stir together flour, cinnamon, baking powder, and soda to blend well.
5. Add oats to creamed mixture along with flour mixture, raisins, and liquid in which raisins were soaked. Mix at medium speed until flour is moistened.
6. Drop by heaping tablespoonfuls onto nonstick cookie sheets or sheets that have been lined with aluminum foil. Press down lightly with fingers dipped in cold water to form circles about 2 inches across. Bake for 10–12 minutes. Transfer from hot cookie sheet to wire rack to cool to room temperature.

Yield: 3 dozen cookies

Nutritive values per 1-cookie serving:	CAL	CHO (gm)	PRO (gm)	FAT (gm)
	74	10	2	3

Food exchanges per 1-cookie serving: ½ BREAD, ½ FAT

Cherry Pie

This is a good cherry pie recipe that I adapted from The New Diabetic Cookbook, *by Mabel Cavaiani (Contemporary Books, 1984).*

> 2   16-ounce cans unsweetened red cherries, drained, liquid reserved
> 1   tablespoon cornstarch
> 18   packages artificial sweetener (Equal)
> ¼   teaspoon almond flavoring
> 1   teaspoon vanilla extract
> ½   teaspoon each ground cinnamon and mace
> 1   prebaked single-crust Lean Pie Crust (recipe follows)

1. Combine 1 cup reserved cherry liquid and cornstarch. Cook and stir over moderate heat until thickened and transparent and the starchy taste is gone. Remove from heat and add sweetener, almond flavoring, vanilla, spices, and cherries. Taste and add more sweetener, if desired. Cool to room temperature.
2. Spread filling evenly in crust. Let set at least 15 minutes. Cut into 8 equal portions.

Yield: 1 9-inch pie (8 servings)

Nutritive values per serving:	CAL	CHO (gm)	PRO (gm)	FAT (gm)
	124	20	2	4

Food exchanges per serving: ⅔ BREAD, 1 FRUIT, 1 FAT

Lean Pie Crust

½ cup sifted unbleached white flour
¼ teaspoon salt
¼ teaspoon double-acting baking powder
¼ cup diet margarine at room temperature

1. Stir flour, salt, and baking powder together. Cut in margarine with fork or pastry blender and continue mixing until no pastry sticks to the sides of the bowl. Shape into a ball. Wrap and refrigerate for an hour or more.
2. Roll the dough out on a floured board. If prebaking, heat oven to 425°F and bake about 12 minutes or until golden.

Yield: 1 single-crust 8- or 9-inch pie shell (8 servings)

Nutritive values per serving:

	CAL	CHO (gm)	PRO (gm)	FAT (gm)
	50	7	1	2

Food exchanges per serving: ½ BREAD, ½ FAT

Quick Banana Cream Pie

If you use the vanilla pudding mix, you might try adding ½ teaspoon extra vanilla for more flavor.

1 Graham Cracker Crust (recipe follows)
1 envelope (.087 ounce) Bird's English Custard (my favorite) *or* 1 4-serving package sugar-free vanilla pudding mix
2 large *or* 3 medium firm-ripe bananas

1. Prepare the pie crust according to the recipe directions and chill.
2. Following the package directions, prepare the custard using artificial sweetener to replace the sugar, or prepare the sugar-free pudding mix.
3. Slice 1½ bananas into the bottom of the pie crust. Pour

pudding or custard over the top. Slice remaining ½ banana and arrange in circles over top. Chill for 2–3 hours.

Yield: 8 servings

Nutritive values per serving of filling:	CAL	CHO (gm)	PRO (gm)	FAT (gm)
	73	12	4	1

Food exchanges per serving of filling: ½ FRUIT, ½ MILK, trace FAT

Total nutritive values per serving:	CAL	CHO (gm)	PRO (gm)	FAT (gm)
	189	30	6	1

Total food exchanges per serving: 1 BREAD, ½ FRUIT, ½ MILK, 1 FAT

Graham Cracker Crust

¾ cup graham cracker crumbs
2 tablespoons wheat germ
⅓ cup diet margarine

Blend crumbs, wheat germ, and margarine thoroughly with a fork or fingers. Press firmly into a nonstick 8- or 9-inch pie plate.

Yield: 1 8- or 9-inch pie crust

Nutritive values per ⅛-crust serving:	CAL	CHO (gm)	PRO (gm)	FAT (gm)
	116	18	2	4

Food exchanges per ⅛-crust serving: 1 BREAD, 1 FAT

Fresh Peach Pie

My mom, Dorothy Rosenberg, sent this lower-calorie recipe and it's great. I've provided the exchanges for the filling in case you want to use a different pastry recipe.

> 2 tablespoons brown sugar
> 4 packets artificial sweetener (equal to 8 teaspoons sugar)
> 1 tablespoon cornstarch
> Juice of ½ lemon
> 1½ cups peeled and mashed fresh peaches
> 3 cups peeled and sliced fresh peaches
> Whole Grain Pastry Shell (recipe follows)

1. Combine sugar, sweetener, and cornstarch in a medium saucepan with juice and mashed peaches. Bring to a boil, reduce heat, and simmer about 5 minutes, until mixture is thickened, stirring constantly. Set aside to cool.

2. Place sliced peaches in pastry shell. Spoon cooled peach mixture over peaches and chill thoroughly.

Yield: 8 servings

Nutritive values per serving of filling:	CAL	CHO (gm)	PRO (gm)	FAT (gm)
	56	14	0	0

Food exchanges per serving of filling: 1½ FRUIT

Total nutritive values per serving:	CAL	CHO (gm)	PRO (gm)	FAT (gm)
	170	27	2	6

Total food exchanges per serving: 1 BREAD, 1½ FRUIT, 1 FAT

Whole Grain Pastry Shell

This pastry shell is very tasty and high in fiber. You could use it with any pie filling.

> ³⁄₄ cup whole wheat pastry flour
> ½ cup quick-cooking oats (not instant)
> 1 tablespoon brown sugar
> 1 teaspoon ground cinnamon
> ½ cup diet margarine, melted
> 2 tablespoons water
>   Vegetable oil

1. Preheat oven to 450°F.
2. Combine flour, oats, sugar, and cinnamon in a small bowl. Combine margarine and water; sprinkle over dry ingredients. Mix with a fork until mixture forms a ball.
3. Coat a 9-inch pie plate with vegetable oil; press whole wheat pastry mixture evenly and firmly into pie plate with lightly floured hands. Bake for 12–15 minutes; cool and fill.

Yield: 1 9-inch pie shell

Nutritive values per ⅛-shell serving:	CAL	CHO (gm)	PRO (gm)	FAT (gm)
	114	13	2	6

Food exchanges per ⅛-shell serving: 1 BREAD, 1 FAT

Applesauce Bran Squares

This recipe from The New Diabetic Cookbook, *by Mabel Cavaiani (Contemporary Books, 1984), is very good and high in fiber.*

 1 cup unbleached white flour
 ⅔ cup Bran Buds, All Bran, or 100% Bran
 ½ cup rolled oats (regular or quick, not instant)
 2 tablespoons brown sugar
 ½ teaspoon baking soda
 1 teaspoon double-acting baking powder
 1 teaspoon ground cinnamon
 ¼ teaspoon ground cloves or nutmeg or mace
 ½ cup (1 stick) diet margarine at room temperature
 2 large egg whites at room temperature
 1 teaspoon vanilla extract
 8 packets artificial sweetener (equal to ⅓ cup sugar)
 ⅓ cup chopped nuts
 1 cup unsweetened applesauce at room temperature

1. Preheat oven to 375°F.
2. Place dry ingredients in mixer bowl and mix at low speed for 1 minute.
3. Add margarine, egg whites, vanilla, sweetener, nuts, and applesauce to flour mixture and mix at medium speed for 1 minute or until blended. Spread evenly in a 9- by 13-inch cake pan that has been greased with margarine. Bake for 25–30 minutes or until it is browned and starts to pull away from the sides of the pan. Cut into 15 squares and serve warm or at room temperature.

Yield: 15 servings

Nutritive values per serving:	CAL	CHO (gm)	PRO (gm)	FAT (gm)
	136	13	3	8

Food exchanges per serving: 1 BREAD, 1½ FAT

Carrot Snack Cake

This recipe has lots of good nutrition and is much lower in fats and sugar than any commercial carrot cake you can buy.

  2 cups whole wheat pastry flour
  1 cup unbleached white flour
  2 teaspoons baking soda
  1 teaspoon double-acting baking powder
  8 ounces nonfat yogurt
  1 cup finely grated carrots
  ½ cup honey
  ½ cup raisins
  ⅓ cup unsweetened crushed pineapple, drained
  2 eggs
  ⅓ cup vegetable oil
  2 tablespoons sesame seeds

1. Preheat oven to 350°F.
2. Combine flours, soda, and baking powder in mixing bowl. Stir well to blend ingredients.
3. Add remaining ingredients except sesame seeds. Beat only to moisten.
4. Spread batter in greased 9- by 13-inch baking pan. Sprinkle on sesame seeds. Bake for about 30 minutes. Cool. Cut into 24 squares.

Yield: 24 squares

Nutritive values per 1-square serving:	CAL	CHO (gm)	PRO (gm)	FAT (gm)
	124	19	3	4

Food exchanges per 1-square serving: 1 BREAD, ½ FRUIT, 1 FAT

Vanilla Cheesecake

1½ envelopes unflavored gelatin
½ cup cold water
1 cup evaporated skim milk
1½ cups low-fat vanilla yogurt
2 cups low-fat cottage cheese
1 teaspoon vanilla extract
12 packets artificial sweetener (Equal)
¼ cup diet margarine, melted
¾ cup graham cracker crumbs

1. In a small saucepan, dissolve gelatin in ½ cup cold water and the evaporated milk. Heat mixture until tiny bubbles form around edge of pan. Stir to dissolve gelatin completely. Let cool to room temperature.
2. Using a blender or food processor, combine yogurt and cottage cheese until smooth. (If using a blender, add yogurt first.)
3. Combine yogurt mixture with the cooled milk. Add vanilla extract and sweetener.
4. Refrigerate filling, stirring occasionally, until thickened.
5. Combine margarine and graham cracker crumbs. Mix well. Press mixture evenly on the bottom of a 9-inch springform pan. Bake 8 minutes at 375°F. Cool on a wire rack.
6. Pour filling into crust, cover, and refrigerate at least 4 hours or until firm.

Variations

1. To reduce the exchanges for a snack, serve half a slice and top it with ⅓ cup strawberries. (Add ½ FRUIT.)
2. Top the whole cheesecake with 1½ cups sliced strawberries *or* 1 8-ounce can unsweetened crushed pineapple, drained. (Add 10 calories and ¼ FRUIT per serving.)
3. Top each full-slice serving with ½ cup Strawberry Sauce (see index for recipe).

Yield: 8 servings

Nutritive values per serving:	CAL	CHO (gm)	PRO (gm)	FAT (gm)
	247	25	12	11

Food exchanges per serving: ½ BREAD, 1 MILK, 2 FAT

Oatmeal Bread

I love homemade bread, and this one is so good that one loaf lasts only about eight hours at my house. If your family likes this bread as much as mine does, you might want to double the recipe. The rising time makes this a little time-consuming, so if you don't work at home, try making it on a weekend. Red-Star makes a "quick-rise" yeast that will rise up to 50 percent faster. Follow the package instructions.

> 1 cup plus 2 tablespoons skim milk
> 2 tablespoons diet margarine
> 2½ tablespoons honey
> 1¼ teaspoons salt
> 1 package (1 scant tablespoon) active dry yeast
> ¼ cup warm water (105–115°F)
> 1 cup rolled oats (regular or quick, not instant)
> 3–3¼ cups unbleached white flour
> Vegetable oil

1. Scald milk and add margarine, honey, and salt, stirring until margarine melts. Let mixture cool to between 105 and 115°F.
2. Combine yeast and warm water in a large bowl; let stand 5 minutes. Add milk mixture, oats, and 2 cups flour; mix well. Stir in enough of the remaining flour to make a soft dough.
3. Turn dough out onto a lightly floured surface; knead until smooth and elastic (about 8–10 minutes). Place dough in a large bowl, coated with a little vegetable oil, turning to grease top. Cover and let rise in a warm place (85°F), free from drafts, 1 hour or until doubled in bulk. Punch dough down, cover, and let dough stand 10 minutes.
4. Turn dough out onto a lightly floured surface. Roll into a 15- by 19-inch rectangle. Roll up, jelly roll fashion, beginning at narrow edge. Pinch seam and ends to-

gether to seal; place roll, seam side down, in a 9- by 5-
by 3-inch loaf pan coated with a little vegetable oil.

5. Cover and let rise 50 minutes or until doubled in bulk.
Bake at 375°F for 40–45 minutes. Remove from pan;
cool on wire rack.

Variation

Add ½ cup currants, soaked in warm water to plump and
drained, at the end of step 2.

Yield: 1 loaf

Nutritive values per ½-inch-slice serving:	CAL	CHO (gm)	PRO (gm)	FAT (gm)
	110	20	3	2

Food exchanges per ½-inch-slice serving:	1 BREAD, ½ FRUIT, ½ FAT

Nutritive values of variation per ½-inch-slice serving:	CAL	CHO (gm)	PRO (gm)	FAT (gm)
	118	22	3	2

Food exchanges of variation per ½-inch-slice serving:	1 BREAD, ½ FRUIT, ½ FAT

Zucchini Bread

This recipe is from The New Diabetic Cookbook, *by Mabel Cavaiani (Contemporary Books, 1984). I use whole wheat pastry flour for added nutrition and fiber.*

- 1 cup unbleached white flour
- ¾ cup whole wheat pastry flour
- 1½ teaspoons ground cinnamon
- ¼ teaspoon salt
- 1 teaspoon baking soda
- ½ teaspoon double-acting baking powder
- 3 large egg whites
- ⅓ cup vegetable oil
- 1½ teaspoons vanilla extract
- 3 packets artificial sweetener (equal to 2 tablespoons sugar)
- 1½ cups well-packed shredded fresh zucchini

1. Preheat oven to 375°F.
2. Place flour, cinnamon, salt, soda, and baking powder in a mixer bowl and mix at low speed to blend well.
3. Place egg whites, oil, vanilla, and sweetener in a cup and mix well with a fork to blend.
4. Add zucchini to flour mixture along with oil mixture and mix at medium speed until well blended and creamy.
5. Pour into 9- by 5- by 3-inch loaf pan that has been greased with diet margarine. Bake for 45 minutes or until a cake tester comes out clean from the center and the bread pulls away from the side of the pan. Cool in the pan for 10 minutes. Turn out onto a wire rack and cool to room temperature.

Yield: 18 ½-inch slices

Nutritive values per ½-inch-slice serving:	CAL	CHO (gm)	PRO (gm)	FAT (gm)
	84	10	2	4

Food exchanges per ½-inch-slice serving: ⅔ BREAD, 1 FAT

9
Dinner

Dinner is traditionally the big family meal in this country. Everyone sits down to a hearty meal of meat and potatoes with a tasty dessert. As we discussed earlier, too much of a good thing is still too much. We've become oversaturated (quite literally) with animal proteins and animal fats. With a diabetic in the family, your attention has turned to low-fat cooking and lower-fat foods, less meat, less sugar, etc., and that's the good side of diabetes.

There is every good reason why your whole family will benefit from your child's diabetic diet. There is no good reason you can't enjoy all the family favorites and create new ones as well. This chapter combines familiar dishes like lasagne, pizza, barbecued chicken, and pot roast with new dishes like Lemon Chicken with Bulgur, Salmon Croquettes, Orange Pork Chops with Rice, and Lean Pastichio. They are all formulated with the diabetic's diet requirements *and* family eating in mind.

Generally, I like to delay desserts to a snack time so that the most nutritious food is served for meals. Even so, I have included a few desserts here, even one that's free food! I've added them as suggestions for several different reasons. Lemon Snow Pudding is free, up to a 2-cup serving! Chocolate Delight is a MILK and could easily replace ½ MILK exchange with dinner. The last few dishes—All-American Cranberry Sauce, Cranberry Relish, etc.—are there for special holiday dinners. If your child is allowed a FRUIT exchange at dinner, there are several recipes in "Snacks" that also count as FRUIT— Frozen Fruit Pops, Orange or Pineapple Sherbert, and Wholesome Brownies.

Once again, don't be limited by the way I've organized the meals. There are many dishes in the "Lunch" chapter that are great for dinner. Use the master list of recipes at the back of the book to design your own menus.

This chapter includes lots of starchy and nonstarchy vegetable dishes with which to tempt your children. The best approach with nutrition in general is to eat a wide variety of foods, so try introducing your family to new taste treats. As I discuss in the introduction to Bulgur Pilaf, try introducing new grain products slowly. Mix them half-and-half with a more familiar grain. Tastes can change, but it takes patience.

Also, instead of concentrating on the vegetables your child doesn't eat, make a list, with your child, of the ones she will eat and serve something each child likes at each meal. For example, my secretary, Judy Garcia, chops up all the salad vegetables and lets each family member choose the contents of his salad bowl—sort of a do-it-yourself salad bar. If some of the more seemingly exotic vegetables like Swiss chard aren't big successes, don't worry. Use the "sneaky vegetable" recipes like Tamale Pie and Vegetable and Meat Loaf.

This chapter begins with salad and pasta main courses. Next there are recipes for poultry, fish, and then meats. Potato, rice, grains, and vegetable dishes follow, and the chapter ends with a few salad dressings, a nonfat gravy, and desserts.

Happy eating!

DINNER MENU IDEAS

You will need to alter these menus to fit your child's diet plan. (Check the index to locate recipes.)

MENU 1

1 cup Gloria's Spaghetti Sauce with 2 meatballs or sausage — 3 medium-fat MEAT, 2½ VEGETABLE, 2 FAT
1 cup pasta — 2 BREAD
1-2 cups Vegetable Salad: lettuce, grated carrots, — 1 or 2 VEGETABLE; ½ FAT

cucumbers, sprouts, etc.,
  with Creamy Vinaigrette
Continental Green Beans   2 VEGETABLE

TOTAL: 2 BREAD, 3 medium-fat MEAT, 5½–6½ VEGETABLE, 2½ FAT

MENU 2

BBQ Chicken   2 lean MEAT, 1 VEGETABLE,
                          ½ FAT
Carrot–Acorn Squash   1 BREAD, 1 VEGETABLE
Steamed Broccoli   1 VEGETABLE
Lemon Snow Pudding   FREE

TOTAL: 1 BREAD, 2 lean MEAT, 3 VEGETABLE, ½ FAT

MENU 3

Tamale Pie   1½ BREAD, 1½ medium-fat MEAT,
                          ½ FAT
Cauliflower Parmesan   1 VEGETABLE, ½ FAT
Baked Spinach   1 VEGETABLE, ½ FAT
Apple Salad (from "Snacks"   1 FRUIT
  chapter)

TOTAL: 1½ BREAD, 1 FRUIT, 1½ medium-fat MEAT, 2 VEGETABLE,
  1½ FAT

MENU 4

Lemon Chicken   3 lean MEAT, ½ FAT
Corn Pudding   1 BREAD, ½ MILK, ½ lean MEAT,
                          1 FAT
Salad with Tangy Buttermilk   2 VEGETABLE
  Dressing
Zucchini Italiano   2 VEGETABLE
Chocolate Delight   ½ MILK, trace FAT

TOTAL: 1 BREAD, 1 MILK, 3½ lean MEAT, 4 VEGETABLE, 1½ FAT

MENU 5

Chicken & Vegetable Stir-Fry   3½ lean MEAT, 2 VEGETABLE
1 cup rice   2 BREAD
Cucumber Salad   ½ VEGETABLE, trace FAT
Pineapple Sherbert (from   ½ FRUIT
  "Snacks" chapter)

TOTAL: 2 BREAD, ½ FRUIT, 3½ lean MEAT, 2½ VEGETABLE, trace
  FAT

DINNER EXCHANGES

Use this list as a quick reference when planning dinner menus. A glance at the right-hand column should give you ideas of what to serve for certain exchanges called for in your child's diet plan. The recipes are listed here in the same order as they appear in the chapter.

Linguine with Red Clam Sauce	2 BREAD, 3 lean MEAT, 1 VEGETABLE
Lasagne with Meat and Vegetables	1½ BREAD, 3 medium-fat MEAT, 2 VEGETABLE, 1½ FAT
Spinach Manicotti	2 BREAD, 1½ medium-fat MEAT, 3 VEGETABLE
Pasta with Tuna and Tomato Sauce	2 BREAD, 2 lean MEAT, 1 VEGETABLE
Whole Wheat Pizza	2 BREAD, 3 medium-fat MEAT, 1 VEGETABLE
Tamale Pie	1½ BREAD, 1½ medium-fat MEAT, ½ FAT
Gloria's Spaghetti Sauce With Meat	2½ VEGETABLE, trace FAT 3 medium-fat MEAT, 2½ VEGETABLE, 2 FAT
Fast Spaghetti Sauce	1½ medium-fat MEAT, 2 VEGETABLE
With Spaghetti Squash	1 BREAD
Chinese Chicken Salad	1½ lean MEAT, 2 VEGETABLE, 2 FAT
Taco Salad	1 BREAD, 1½ high-fat MEAT, 2 VEGETABLE
Lemon Chicken	3 lean MEAT, ½ FAT
Chicken and Vegetable Stir-Fry	3½ lean MEAT, 2 VEGETABLE
Chicken Cacciatore	3 lean MEAT, 2 VEGETABLE, ½ FAT
Lemon Chicken with Bulgur	3 BREAD, 3 medium-fat MEAT
Foiled Chicken	3 lean MEAT, 1 VEGETABLE
Orange Chicken	3 lean MEAT

BBQ Chicken   2 lean MEAT, 1 VEGETABLE,
                               ½ FAT

Oven-Fried Chicken   2 BREAD, 3½ lean MEAT,
                               trace FAT

Peanut Butter Chicken   2 lean MEAT, 1½ VEGETABLE,
                               1 FAT

Chicken Pizzaiola   1½ BREAD, 4½ lean MEAT,
                               3 VEGETABLE, 1½ FAT

Chicken Cordon Bleu   ⅓ BREAD, 4 lean MEAT, ½ FAT

Brunswick Stew   2 BREAD, 2½ lean MEAT

Turkey Loaf   3 lean MEAT, 1½ VEGETABLE

Roast Stuffed Turkey   5 lean MEAT

Stuffing with Whole Wheat   1⅔ BREAD
  Bread
  With ½ Bread and ½   2 BREAD, trace FAT
  Cornbread
  With Cornbread   2 BREAD, ½ FAT

Turkey Burgers   ⅓ BREAD, 2 lean MEAT

Turkey Tetrazzini   2 BREAD, 2 lean MEAT, trace FAT

Seafood Stew   5½ lean MEAT, 1 VEGETABLE

Oven "French-Fried" Scallops   ⅔ BREAD, 3 lean MEAT

Saucy Scallops   ½ BREAD, 4 lean MEAT

Foiled Fish Fillets   4½ lean MEAT

Oven Fish Fillets   ⅓ MILK, 3 lean MEAT

Salmon Croquettes   1 BREAD, 3 lean MEAT

Mustard Sauce   ½ FAT

Lean Pastichio   1 BREAD, 2 medium-fat MEAT,
                               1 VEGETABLE
  With Feta Cheese   1 BREAD, 2½ medium-fat MEAT,
                               1 VEGETABLE

Beef and Tomato Stir-Fry   1 BREAD, 3 lean MEAT,
                               2 VEGETABLE

Oriental Flank Steak   4 lean MEAT, ½ FAT

Pot Roast   1 BREAD, 4½ medium-fat MEAT

Beef and Snow Peas   2 lean MEAT, 1½ VEGETABLE,
                               ½ FAT

Vegetable and Meat Loaf	3 lean MEAT, 1 VEGETABLE
Swiss Steak	½ BREAD, 4 lean MEAT, 1 VEGETABLE, ½ FAT
Superb Oven Stew	2 BREAD, 4 lean MEAT
Veal Scaloppine	⅓ BREAD, 3 lean MEAT, ½ FAT
Osso Buco	3 lean MEAT, 1 VEGETABLE
Veal Chops with Raspberry Vinegar	3 lean MEAT, ½ FAT
Greek Lamb Chops	3 lean MEAT
Lovely Lamb Stew	1 BREAD, 4 lean MEAT
Baked Lamb Chops	1 FRUIT, 3 lean MEAT, ½ FAT
Orange Pork Chops with Rice	1½ BREAD, 1 FRUIT, 4 lean MEAT
Noodle Kugel	2 BREAD, 1 FRUIT, 1 lean MEAT
Red Beans and Rice	3 BREAD, 1 lean MEAT, 1 VEGETABLE
Rice and Vegetable Casserole	1 BREAD, 1½ VEGETABLE
Bulgur Pilaf	2 BREAD
Oven "French Fries"	1 BREAD, ½ FAT
Potato-Bean Patties	1 BREAD, 1 medium-fat MEAT
Potato Kugel	1 BREAD, trace FAT
Stuffed Yams	2 BREAD, ½ FRUIT
Puffed Sweet Potatoes	2 BREAD
Sweet Potatoes and Bananas	1 BREAD, 1 FRUIT
Carrot–Acorn Squash	1 BREAD, 1 VEGETABLE
Corn Pudding	1 BREAD, ½ MILK, ½ lean MEAT, 1 FAT
Squash with Apples	1 BREAD, 1 FRUIT, trace FAT
Oven-Fried Squash	½ BREAD, 1 VEGETABLE, trace FAT
Cauliflower or Broccoli Parmesan	1 VEGETABLE, ½ FAT
Sesame Broccoli Variation	1½ VEGETABLE, ½ FAT 2½ VEGETABLE, ½ FAT

Tart Red Cabbage	1 FRUIT, 1 VEGETABLE
Sautéed Cabbage	1 VEGETABLE
Fruit Spiced Carrots	1 VEGETABLE
Cucumber Salad	½ VEGETABLE, trace FAT
Continental Green Beans	2 VEGETABLE
Baked Spinach	1 VEGETABLE, ½ FAT
Stir-Fry Squash	1 VEGETABLE, ½ FAT
Zucchini Italiano	2 VEGETABLE
Swiss Chard Sauté	1½ VEGETABLE, ½ FAT
Mashed Turnips	1½ VEGETABLE
Hash Brown Turnips	1½ VEGETABLE
Chinese Vegetables	1½ VEGETABLE
Skillet Vegetables	½ high-fat MEAT, 2 VEGETABLE
Popovers	1 BREAD, 1 FAT
No-Calorie Dressing	FREE up to ½ cup
Tangy Buttermilk Dressing	FREE up to ⅓ cup
Mock Thousand Island Dressing	½ BREAD
Creamy Vinaigrette	½ FAT
Low-Calorie Mayonnaise	½ lean MEAT, ½ FAT
Gravy from Meat Drippings	FREE
Lemon Snow Pudding	FREE up to 2 cups
Chocolate Delight	½ MILK, trace FAT
Chocolate Sauce	¼ MILK, trace FAT
All-American Cranberry Sauce	½ FRUIT
Cranberry Relish	½ FRUIT; up to 4 tablespoons FREE
Cranberry Mold	1 FRUIT, ½ FAT
Cran-Apple Crisp	½ BREAD, 1½ FRUIT, 1 FAT
Easy Sugarless Pumpkin Pie	1½ BREAD, ½ MILK, 1 FAT

Recipes

PASTA PLUS

Most of us have had the mistaken notion that pasta is a fattening filler food, laden with calories and not terribly nutritious. Nothing could be further from the truth. Pasta is a nourishing food that fills you up before you eat more calories than you need. Pasta is also an ideal basic food for diabetics since it is very low on the glycemic index; therefore, it does not cause blood sugar to rise very much after a meal.

A 1-cup serving of cooked pasta weighs about 5 ounces, has only 200 calories, and has half the calories of a steak the same size. The 1-cup serving counts as 2 BREAD. The problem with pasta is that we Americans tend to drown it in rich cream and butter-laden sauces. Even ⅔ cup plain canned tomato sauce counts as 1 BREAD. The secret is to keep the fat content very low and add fiber to the sauces. I use canned whole tomatoes and puree them very briefly, leaving chunks of tomato still intact. Better yet, break up the tomatoes by hand. Sneaky vegetables—chopped onion, spinach, broccoli, and grated carrots—add important fiber to the sauce.

If your child loves pasta but is allowed only 2 BREAD at dinner, try trading the carbohydrates from another exchange like FRUIT or MILK. The 10 grams of carbohydrate in a FRUIT would count as ⅔ BREAD, hence another ⅓ cup pasta. A MILK is 12 grams, which would be almost the same as 1 BREAD (15 grams carbohydrate), allowing another ½-cup serving. I discuss trading exchanges in detail in Part III: "The Copebook."

You do not need to add salt to the water in which you cook your pasta. If no salt is added, a 1-cup serving of pasta contains less than 10 milligrams of sodium. Pasta also contains reasonable amounts of thiamine, riboflavin, niacin, and iron and 5 grams of protein per 1-cup serving.

Pasta comes dried or fresh, in many colors, in dozens of different shapes and sizes, and from many different types of flour. Pasta from durum wheat semolina cooks up firm and slightly chewy (al dente—"to the tooth") if not over-cooked. There are new high-protein pastas available. They contain approximately 13 grams of protein per 1-cup serving, the same amount you would get from 2 ounces of meat. Pastas are a good idea for children who are fussy eaters. I've never met a child who didn't like pasta. You can serve it with a tomato sauce with sneaky vegetables (Gloria's Spaghetti Sauce) or plain with a glass of milk and carrot sticks, for instance, and know your child has had a nutritious meal.

Whole wheat pasta is available in health food stores and some large supermarkets. It has more fiber, vitamins, and minerals than regular pasta, but the taste and texture are much different. Try mixing the two, but cook them separately. Whole wheat pasta can get mushy if cooked as long as regular pasta.

You can now buy fresh pasta—pasta that has not been dried. You don't necessarily get a superior product, although you'll pay a premium price. Also, fresh pasta contains more water than dried, so the price per pound cannot be compared directly. A pound of fresh pasta does not go as far as a pound of dried. Fresh pasta absorbs sauce more readily, so it works best with light sauces. It cooks very quickly—in 2–6 minutes as compared to 8–20 minutes for dried pasta.

Cook pasta in a large pot with 4–6 quarts of water per pound of pasta. The more water, the less gummy the pasta will be. Add the pasta to the rapidly boiling water in batches over a span of no more than 1 minute. Drain in a colander and do not rinse it unless it's to be used for a cold salad.

Linguine with Red Clam Sauce

If your child likes clams still in their shells, use fresh clams. If not, use canned clams. I first had this years ago in Italy, prepared by the waiter at the table after I told him I love clams.

1 clove garlic, minced or pressed
1 tablespoon extra-virgin olive oil
¼ cup white wine
1 16-ounce can tomatoes
2 tablespoons tomato paste
1 teaspoon basil leaves
½ teaspoon oregano leaves
2 tablespoons chopped fresh parsley
¼ teaspoon freshly ground pepper
Juice of ½ lemon
1 dozen Little Neck clams *or* 2 10-ounce cans clams, whole or chopped
8 ounces dry linguine, cooked al dente

1. In large skillet, sauté garlic in oil over medium heat until softened, 2 or 3 minutes. Do not let it brown.
2. Add remaining ingredients except clams and linguine and simmer over low heat for 20–25 minutes. Stir and break up tomatoes.
3. Add clams, whole in shells or canned (with juice). Cover and steam whole clams for 10 minutes or until clams open or for 3 or 4 minutes if using canned clams.
4. Toss with hot, drained pasta and serve.

Yield: 4 1½-cup servings

Nutritive values per 1½-cup serving:	CAL	CHO (gm)	PRO (gm)	FAT (gm)
	289	35	26	5

Food exchanges per 1½-cup serving: 2 BREAD, 3 lean MEAT, 1 VEGETABLE

Lasagne with Meat and Vegetables

½ pound lean ground beef
4 sweet Italian sausages, removed from casings (about ½ pound)
1 bunch spinach (approximately 1 pound)
1 large stalk broccoli (about ½ pound)
¼ cup water
½ recipe Gloria's Spaghetti Sauce without meat (about 6 cups) (see index for recipe)
8 ounces lasagne noodles
1 cup low-fat cottage cheese
1 cup ricotta cheese
2 eggs, beaten
¼ cup Parmesan cheese
¼ cup minced fresh parsley
1 cup shredded part-skim mozzarella cheese

1. Preheat oven to 375°F.
2. Fry beef and sausage in large skillet over medium heat until well browned but still soft. Drain well on paper towels in a colander. Wipe all drippings from pan.
3. Clean spinach, remove stems, and shred spinach with a sharp knife, cutting across the leaf. Cut tough ends off the bottom of the broccoli. Peel the stems. Chop the flowerets and stems. Put the spinach and broccoli in skillet, add ¼ cup water, cover, and steam over medium heat for 5 minutes.
4. Add the meat and vegetables to the sauce and simmer for 30–45 minutes.
5. Meanwhile, cook the lasagne noodles a few at a time in lots of boiling water until al dente. Drain and spread on wax paper.
6. Combine the cottage cheese, ricotta, eggs, Parmesan cheese, and parsley.
7. When sauce is ready, spread ½ cup sauce in the bottom of a 13- by 9-inch baking dish. Next, put in a layer of noodles, ½ the cottage cheese mixture, ½ the mozzarella, 1 cup sauce, another layer of noodles, the remain-

ing cottage cheese mixture, 1 cup sauce, remaining noodles, 1 cup sauce, and the remaining mozzarella. Reserve extra sauce to pass separately.

8. Bake for 30–40 minutes until cheese is bubbling. Remove from oven and allow to stand 20 minutes before cutting. Cut into 10 equal portions.

Yield: 10 1½-cup servings

Nutritive values per 1½-cup serving:	CAL	CHO (gm)	PRO (gm)	FAT (gm)
	423	26	28	23

Food exchanges per 1½-cup serving:

1½ BREAD, 3 medium-fat MEAT, 1 VEGETABLE, 1½ FAT

Spinach Manicotti

I've found the easiest way to stuff the shells is to use a pastry bag with a wide tip. If you don't have a pastry bag, slit one side of each shell with a sharp knife, open it, and fill. Place the cut side down in the baking dish and no one will be the wiser! If you use a spaghetti sauce from a jar, look for one with no added sugar.

  10 manicotti shells
    2 10-ounce packages frozen chopped spinach *or* 2 bunches (approximately 1 pound each) fresh
    1 16-ounce carton low-fat cottage cheese, drained, *or* 1 16-ounce carton ricotta cheese
  ⅓ cup grated Parmesan cheese
  ¼ teaspoon ground nutmeg
      Freshly ground pepper, to taste
  ¼ teaspoon extra-virgin olive oil
    4 cups meatless spaghetti sauce (preferably homemade)
  ¼ cup chopped fresh parsley

1. Preheat oven to 350°F.
2. Cook manicotti shells according to package directions, omitting salt; drain and set aside.
3. Cook spinach according to package directions, omitting salt. Drain, place on paper towels, and squeeze until barely moist. Or wash fresh spinach, remove stems, and shred across leaf. Steam for 5 minutes and drain thoroughly.
4. Combine spinach, cottage cheese, Parmesan cheese, nutmeg, and pepper. Stuff manicotti shells with spinach mixture and arrange in a 13- by 9-inch baking dish wiped with olive oil.
5. Pour spaghetti sauce over manicotti. Bake for 45 minutes. Sprinkle with parsley.

Yield: 5 servings (2 manicotti each)

Nutritive values per serving:	CAL	CHO (gm)	PRO (gm)	FAT (gm)
	350	44	21	10

Food exchanges per serving: 2 BREAD, 1½ medium-fat MEAT, 3 VEGETABLE

Pasta with Tuna and Tomato Sauce

I tasted this in Italy, where it was called Spaghetti with Tuna Sauce, and it was delicious. This is my adaptation of it.

- 2 cloves garlic, minced or pressed
- 1 tablespoon extra-virgin olive oil
- 1 anchovy fillet
- ½ medium onion, chopped
- 1 16-ounce can Italian tomatoes, pureed in blender briefly
- 1 teaspoon basil leaves
- ¼ teaspoon ground allspice
- ¼ teaspoon freshly ground pepper
- 1 7-ounce can tuna packed in water, drained and flaked
- ¼ cup minced fresh parsley
- 8 ounces dry pasta, such as rigatoni or rotini (corkscrews) or shells, cooked al dente

1. In large skillet, sauté garlic in oil. Mash anchovy and stir in. Cook for 1 minute.
2. Add onion, tomatoes, and seasonings. Heat to boiling, reduce heat, and simmer for 20 minutes, covered.
3. Add tuna and parsley. Simmer for 10 minutes more.
4. Toss with hot, drained pasta and serve.

Yield: 4 1½-cup servings

Nutritive values per 1½-cup serving:	CAL	CHO (gm)	PRO (gm)	FAT (gm)
	269	35	21	5

Food exchanges per 1½-cup serving: 2 BREAD, 2 lean MEAT, 1 VEGETABLE

Whole Wheat Pizza

Here's a dinner project in which the whole family can participate. You can use your own homemade sauce or a commercial sauce in a jar. If it's not thick, simmer it for 20–25 minutes to reduce and thicken. Measure after reducing.

½ cup warm water (105–115°F)
1 tablespoon extra-virgin olive oil
1 teaspoon sugar
½ teaspoon salt
½ package (about 1 teaspoon) dry yeast
¾ cup unbleached white flour
¾ cup whole wheat flour
  Olive oil
½ pound lean ground beef
1 cup thick tomato sauce (preferably homemade or low-sodium)
1 cup (4 ounces) shredded mozzarella cheese
2 tablespoons grated Parmesan cheese
  Crushed hot red pepper (optional)

1. Combine water, 1 tablespoon olive oil, sugar, and salt in a medium mixing bowl. Sprinkle yeast over mixture, stirring until dissolved. Gradually add flours, mixing well after each addition.
2. Turn dough out onto a lightly floured surface and knead about 4 minutes or until smooth and elastic. Shape into a ball and place in a bowl coated with a little olive oil, turning to grease top. Cover and let rise in a warm place (85°F), free from drafts, 1 hour or until doubled in bulk.
3. Coat a 12-inch pizza pan with ½ teaspoon olive oil and set aside. Punch dough down. Lightly coat hands with oil and pat dough evenly into pizza pan. Bake at 425°F for 5 minutes.
4. Cook ground beef in a skillet over medium heat until meat is browned, stirring to crumble. Drain well on paper towels.

5. Spread 1 cup tomato sauce evenly over pizza crust, leaving a ½-inch border around edges. Sprinkle mozzarella cheese over top. Sprinkle meat over mozzarella, then sprinkle on Parmesan cheese and red pepper flakes. Bake at 425°F 15 minutes, until cheese is bubbling.

Yield: 1 large pizza (4 servings, 2 wedges each)

Nutritive values per 2-wedge serving:	CAL	CHO (gm)	PRO (gm)	FAT (gm)
	397	36	25	17

Food exchanges per 2-wedge serving:

2 BREAD, 3 medium-fat MEAT, 1 VEGETABLE

Tamale Pie

This should be subtitled "with more sneaky vegetables."
Using less meat and more vegetables is a great way to
increase fiber and lower fat. Cook the pinto or red beans
fresh. It doesn't take that long. Cover them with water
and simmer for 1½–2 hours. You can use canned if you
must. Brennan loved this, and Robin didn't. You can't
win 'em all!

Filling
1 pound lean ground beef
2 tablespoons chopped capers
2 cloves garlic, minced or pressed
1 medium onion, chopped
2 medium green peppers, chopped fine
1 tablespoon extra-virgin olive oil
2 tablespoons tomato paste
1 teaspoon ground cumin
2 tablespoons chili powder
½ cup water
3 cups cooked pinto or red beans (1½ cups dried before cooking) *or* 1½ 16-ounce cans, drained and rinsed
1 cup fresh or frozen corn kernels
¼ cup sliced green olives
¼ cup minced fresh parsley

Crust
1 cup stone-ground yellow cornmeal
2 tablespoons unbleached white flour
1½ teaspoons baking powder
1 egg, beaten
½ cup skim milk
1 tablespoon vegetable oil
¼ cup grated sharp Cheddar cheese

1. Preheat oven to 375°F.
2. Sauté beef in large skillet until browned, stirring as it cooks to break up meat. Drain meat thoroughly and spread in the bottom of a 2-quart casserole.

3. In the same skillet, sauté capers, garlic, onion, and peppers in olive oil until softened, 5 minutes or so, over medium heat.

4. Stir in tomato paste, cumin, chili powder, water, beans, corn, olives, and parsley. Stir to combine and cook until mixture is heated through, 10 minutes or so. Pour this mixture on top of meat in casserole and spread evenly.

5. In medium bowl, combine cornmeal, flour, baking powder, egg, milk, and vegetable oil. Spread on top of bean mixture and top with grated cheese.

6. Bake for 25–30 minutes, until bubbly hot and dough is golden brown.

Yield: 10 1-cup servings

Nutritive values per 1-cup serving:	CAL	CHO (gm)	PRO (gm)	FAT (gm)
	239	22	13	11

Food exchanges per 1-cup serving:

1½ BREAD, 1½ medium-fat MEAT, ½ FAT

PASTA SAUCES

Gloria's Spaghetti Sauce (Meatless or with Meat)

My dad is a very good cook, and he taught me to respect well-spiced food. This is an adaptation of his recipe, and I always get compliments on it. The addition of aniseed (tastes like licorice) is the secret.

1 tablespoon olive oil
3 cloves garlic, minced very fine
1 large onion, chopped fine
3 carrots, shredded
¼ pound fresh mushrooms, chopped (optional)
½ cup chopped fresh parsley
2 tablespoons basil leaves
½ teaspoon oregano leaves
1 tablespoon aniseed, crushed (use 2 tablespoons if no meat is used)
1½ cups or more dry red wine (Burgundy or Chianti)
2 28-ounce cans whole tomatoes
1 12-ounce can tomato paste

1. Heat olive oil in heavy Dutch oven over medium-low heat. Add garlic and sauté for a few minutes—don't let it brown. Add onion, carrots, mushrooms, parsley, basil, oregano, aniseed, and red wine. Simmer for 10 minutes.
2. Meanwhile, run the tomatoes through a blender or food processor, then add to skillet along with the tomato paste.
3. Cover and let simmer 3–4 hours. Stir several times each hour. Add more wine if too thick.

Yield: 12 cups

Nutritive values per 1-cup serving:	CAL	CHO (gm)	PRO (gm)	FAT (gm)
	69	12	3	1

Food exchanges per 1-cup serving: 2½ VEGETABLE, trace FAT

(It can be counted as VEGETABLE *or* BREAD. It may affect the blood sugar like a BREAD.)

Variation
To make meat sauce, use the same ingredients and directions above, but use only 1 tablespoon aniseed.

8 sweet Italian sausages (approximately 1 pound)
2 pounds lean ground beef
¼ cup wheat germ
¼ cup Parmesan cheese
1 egg
2 tablespoons Worcestershire sauce
   Freshly ground pepper
½ teaspoon oregano leaves

1. Cut each Italian sausage into 4 pieces and brown in heavy skillet. Drain well on paper towels to cut down on grease. Wipe out skillet.
2. Mix remaining ingredients into meatballs the same size as sausage pieces (approximately 1 inch in diameter) and brown in skillet. Drain well.
3. Add sausages and meatballs to sauce after first hour of simmering.

Yield: 12 cups

Nutritive values per 1-cup serving:	CAL	CHO (gm)	PRO (gm)	FAT (gm)
	386	13	25	26

Food exchanges per 1-cup serving: 3 medium-fat MEAT, 2½ VEGETABLE, 2 FAT *or* ⅔ BREAD, 3 medium-fat MEAT, 2 FAT

Fast Spaghetti Sauce with Spaghetti Squash

Here's a quick sauce to make in the microwave. The spaghetti squash is very much like spaghetti, and it has fewer calories plus good fiber. Toss the squash strands with a little sauce before serving and pass extra sauce separately. This makes a very low-calorie, filling main dish when served with Spaghetti Squash. You might also make some pasta the first time, in case the newness of the squash doesn't enjoy instant success with all your family members!

1 pound lean ground beef
1 medium onion, chopped
½ cup chopped celery
¾ cup chopped green pepper
2 carrots, grated
¼ cup chopped fresh parsley
1 clove garlic, minced or pressed
1 teaspoon oregano leaves
1 teaspoon basil leaves
1 tablespoon aniseed, crushed
2 16-ounce cans whole tomatoes, pureed
1 6-ounce can tomato paste
¼ cup red wine

1. Place ground beef in a hard plastic colander. Place vegetables through garlic on top of meat. Place colander over a casserole dish.
2. Microwave on high for 6 minutes, stirring after 3 minutes. Discard any fat that cooks out.
3. Add remaining ingredients to meat and vegetables, place in a 3-quart casserole, and mix well.
4. Cook on high for 10 minutes. Stir and continue cooking 30–35 minutes on simmer.
5. Serve with Spaghetti Squash (see following recipe) or pasta.

Yield: 8 1-cup servings

	CAL	CHO (gm)	PRO (gm)	FAT (gm)
Nutritive values per 1-cup serving:	156	9	12	8

Food exchanges per 1-cup
serving:

1 BREAD, 1½ medium-fat
MEAT, 2 VEGETABLE

Spaghetti Squash

1 large spaghetti squash (approximately
5½–6 pounds)

1. Pierce the squash with a knife and place on a paper
   towel.
2. Cook in microwave on high for 15 minutes. Turn about
   4 times while it is cooking. Or you can cut it in half
   lengthwise, remove seeds, place cut sides down on a
   baking sheet, and bake for 30–40 minutes, until
   tender, at 350°F. When done, knife should insert
   easily.
3. Let it stand 3 minutes after cooking.
4. Cut in half, remove seeds, and pull the strands free
   with two serving forks.

Variation
If desired, toss squash strands with 2 tablespoons diet
margarine (add 1 FAT per serving).

Yield: Approximately 5–6 servings

	CAL	CHO (gm)	PRO (gm)	FAT (gm)
Nutritive values per 1-cup serving:	68	15	2	0

Food exchanges per 1-cup
serving:

1 BREAD

MAIN COURSE SALADS

Chinese Chicken Salad

My mom also gave me this recipe. It takes a bit of work, but it's worth it. The hoisin sauce is available in Oriental markets and some supermarkets. Most large supermarkets carry the dark sesame oil and rice vinegar. If not, you can get it at an Oriental market. It adds a very special flavor!

2 chicken breast halves, skinned
Water or stock
2 green onions, cut up
2 slices peeled fresh gingerroot
2 teaspoons dark sesame oil
1 slice peeled fresh gingerroot, minced
2 tablespoons hoisin sauce
2 tablespoons rice vinegar
1 small head iceberg lettuce, shredded
2 tablespoons minced fresh parsley or cilantro
2 green onions, cut into 2-inch lengths and shredded
2 tablespoons sesame seeds
¼ pound Chinese pea pods, cut julienne or into diagonal strips
1 tablespoon peanut oil
1 teaspoon dark sesame oil
1 tablespoon soy sauce

1. Poach chicken breasts in water or stock to cover with 2 green onions and 2 ginger slices. Bring to a simmer over medium heat, lower heat, and simmer for 10 minutes. Turn breasts over and let stand 15 minutes.
2. When chicken is cooled, heat 2 teaspoons sesame oil in wok or large skillet over medium-high heat. When hot, add minced ginger. Cook until browned, a few minutes, then remove ginger and discard.
3. Shred chicken into long thin strands and add it to oil

in wok. Stir over medium-high heat for 1 or 2 minutes.
Add hoisin sauce and vinegar. Remove from heat.
4. Combine lettuce, parsley or cilantro, 2 green onions,
sesame seeds, and pea pods. Toss and add shredded
chicken. Add peanut oil, 1 teaspoon sesame oil, and soy
sauce. Toss to mix well. Serve immediately.

Yield: 4 1½-cup servings

Nutritive values per 1½-cup serving:	CAL	CHO (gm)	PRO (gm)	FAT (gm)
	231	9	15	15

Food exchanges per 1½-cup
serving:

1½ lean MEAT, 2 VEGETABLE,
2 FAT

Taco Salad

Taco Salad, like Chinese Chicken Salad (recipe follows), is a good one-dish meal (if your kids eat salad!). If you like a little more moisture, try a little extra sprinkling of lemon juice or wine vinegar.

- 1 cup low-calorie Italian dressing
- 1 tablespoon chili powder
- 1 teaspoon ground cumin
- 1 pound lean ground beef, browned, drained, and cooled
- 2 cups cooked pinto beans
- 2 tomatoes, chopped
- 1 small head lettuce, shredded
- 4 green onions, chopped
- 1 green pepper, chopped
- 1 cup chopped Homemade Tortilla Chips (see index) or commercial taco chips
- 1 cup grated Cheddar cheese

1. Mix dressing, chili powder, and cumin with beef.
2. Place all other ingredients in a large bowl. Add beef and toss gently. *Or* layer the ingredients, with lettuce on the bottom, followed by beans, onions, tomatoes, peppers, and meat, and top with chips and cheese.

Yield: 8 1¼-cup servings

Nutritive values per 1½-cup serving:	CAL	CHO (gm)	PRO (gm)	FAT (gm)
	268	14	17	16

Food exchanges per 1½-cup serving:

1 BREAD, 1½ high-fat MEAT, 2 VEGETABLE

POULTRY
Chicken

I've included lots of chicken recipes. Chicken is versatile, appeals to almost all children and adults, and is a relatively inexpensive animal protein source. All these recipes use skinned chicken, which saves lots of calories and fat per serving.

Lemon Chicken

This is always a great success with my boys. They love the lemony flavor. I've marinated this as long as 48 hours because of last-minute changes in dinner plans, and it was even tastier!

> 4   chicken breast halves, skinned and boned
>   Juice of 2 lemons
> 1   tablespoon unsalted butter
> ½   cup dry white wine

1. Flatten chicken with a tenderizer or mallet to about ¼-inch thickness. Pour lemon juice over and marinate in refrigerator at least 4 hours.
2. Melt butter in a skillet over medium heat. Sauté breasts for 5 minutes on each side. Remove and place on hot platter to keep warm.
3. Pour wine into skillet, stirring. Let boil for a few minutes, then pour over the chicken.

Variation:
Add 1 teaspoon ground cumin to the lemon juice.

Yield: 4 servings

Nutritive values per serving:	CAL	CHO (gm)	PRO (gm)	FAT (gm)
	192	0	21	12
Food exchanges per serving:	3 lean MEAT, ½ FAT			

Chicken and Vegetable Stir-Fry

This is quick and easy. You can make the marinade in the morning, put the rice on 30 minutes before dinner, and then cut the vegetables and start cooking.

2 tablespoons water
3 tablespoons rice vinegar
2 tablespoons soy sauce (preferably reduced-sodium)
1 tablespoon cream sherry
1 clove garlic, minced or pressed
1 thin slice peeled gingerroot, minced, *or*
½ teaspoon dried ginger
2 green onions, with tops, sliced
1 pound boneless chicken breasts, skinned and cut into thin strips
2 teaspoons sesame oil
1 cup celery, sliced diagonally
1 cup carrots, sliced diagonally
1 cup broccoli, flowerets and stems, peeled and sliced
1 cup Chinese pea pods, stem ends snipped
1 tablespoon sesame seeds

1. In a glass dish, combine water, vinegar, soy sauce, sherry, garlic, ginger, onions, and chicken and refrigerate for at least 2 hours (the longer, the better).
2. Drain chicken and reserve marinade.
3. In a large skillet or wok, heat sesame oil over medium-high heat until hot. Add chicken and cook, stirring constantly, until chicken loses its pink color. Remove chicken.
4. Add celery, carrots, and broccoli and cook, stirring, for 3 minutes. Add pea pods and marinade and cover. Let vegetables steam for 2–3 minutes.
5. Add chicken and sesame seeds and stir to combine. Vegetables should be crisp-tender, pea pods still bright green. Serve with Chinese or Korean rice, if available.

Yield: 4 1¼-cup servings

Nutritive values per 1¼-cup serving:	CAL	CHO (gm)	PRO (gm)	FAT (gm)
	270	10	26	14

Food exchanges per 1¼-cup serving:

3½ lean MEAT, 2 VEGETABLE

Chicken Cacciatore

This dish is traditionally made with whole chicken pieces. That adds a lot of fat and is messy to eat. My boys liked this much better with the boneless breasts. The recipe is courtesy of Joe Gallison, the fine actor who played my husband on "Days of Our Lives."

6 boneless chicken breast halves, skinned
1 tablespoon olive oil
2 cloves garlic, minced
1 medium onion, chopped
1 8-ounce can tomato sauce
2 16-ounce cans tomatoes
2 teaspoons basil leaves
1 teaspoon oregano leaves
1 teaspoon rosemary leaves
¼ teaspoon freshly ground pepper
¼ cup red wine
2 green peppers, cut into strips
¼ pound fresh mushrooms, sliced

1. Sauté breasts in olive oil a few minutes per side in a large skillet over medium heat.
2. Add all remaining ingredients to skillet. Break up the tomatoes with a wooden spoon. Cover and simmer for 40 minutes.

Yield: 6 servings

Nutritive values per serving:	CAL	CHO (gm)	PRO (gm)	FAT (gm)
	239	11	24	11

Food exchanges per serving:

3 lean MEAT, 2 VEGETABLE, ½ FAT

Lemon Chicken with Bulgur

This delicious high-fiber dish is from Jane Brody's Good
Food Book. *You can make it with kasha (buckwheat
groats) instead of bulgur. I also like it with extra lemon
or you can serve it with lemon wedges. The servings will
include ½ cup bulgur per person.*

2 teaspoons butter or margarine
2 teaspoons olive or peanut oil
1 3½-pound broiler-fryer, skinned and cut
   into serving pieces
   Salt to taste (optional)
   Freshly ground pepper to taste
3 medium onions, chopped (1½–2 cups)
2 cloves garlic, minced (2 teaspoons)
1½ cups bulgur
½ teaspoon ground cardamom
½ teaspoon ground coriander
½ teaspoon ground cumin
   Grated zest and juice of 1 lemon
3 cups boiling chicken broth

1. Preheat oven to 350°F.
2. In a large skillet, heat the butter or margarine and the
   oil, add the chicken, and brown the pieces on all sides.
   Season the chicken with salt and pepper and transfer
   it to a large casserole.
3. Add the onions and garlic to the skillet and cook,
   stirring, until the onions are translucent.
4. Add the bulgur to the skillet, stirring to coat it and
   brown it lightly.
5. Add the cardamom, coriander, cumin, lemon zest, and
   lemon juice to the bulgur mixture, mixing the ingredients well. Spoon the bulgur on top of the chicken.
6. Pour the boiling broth over the chicken and bulgur.
   Cover the casserole and bake for 1 hour or until the
   chicken is tender.

Yield: 6 servings

Nutritive values per serving (3 ounces chicken and ½ cup bulgur):	CAL	CHO (gm)	PRO (gm)	FAT (gm)
	341	44	21	9

Food exchanges per serving
(3 ounces chicken and ½ cup
bulgur): 3 BREAD, 3 medium-fat MEAT

Foiled Chicken

Multiply this recipe by as many servings as you need for your family. No pans to clean!

1 tablespoon chopped fresh dill, parsley, or basil *or* 1 teaspoon dried
1 clove garlic, minced
1 boneless chicken breast half, skinned and cut into 4 pieces
Freshly ground black pepper
½ cup broccoli flowerets, sliced carrots, or cauliflower flowerets
½ lemon

1. Preheat oven to 350°F.
2. Cut a piece of foil (about 12 inches) into large heart shape.
3. Mix herbs and garlic together.
4. Arrange chicken pieces on foil. Do not overlap pieces.
5. Sprinkle herb mixture and black pepper to taste over chicken.
6. Arrange broccoli on top of chicken.
7. Slice lemon and arrange on top of broccoli.
8. Seal package by crimping edges.
9. Place on baking sheet and bake for 30 minutes.
10. Transfer to dinner plate. Sit down, break into packet, and inhale.

Yield: 1 serving

Nutritive values per serving:	CAL	CHO (gm)	PRO (gm)	FAT (gm)
	190	5	23	9

Food exchanges per serving: 3 lean MEAT, 1 VEGETABLE

Orange Chicken

This is delicious and elegant enough for company.

- 1 cup unsweetened orange juice
- 2 tablespoons peeled and minced fresh gingerroot
- 2 teaspoons sesame oil
- 2 tablespoons Dijon mustard
- 1 tablespoon grated orange zest
- 1 tablespoon grated lemon zest
- 4 whole cloves garlic
- 6 boneless chicken breast halves, skinned and boned
- ½ cup chicken broth (preferably homemade)
  Freshly ground pepper (optional)

1. Combine first 7 ingredients in blender or food processor and whirl for 15 seconds. Pour over chicken in a shallow baking pan. Cover with plastic wrap and refrigerate overnight.
2. Preheat oven to 325°F. Remove chicken breasts from marinade, reserving marinade. Sauté breasts in chicken broth 3–4 minutes per side, over medium heat in a large skillet.
3. Transfer breasts to baking pan. Cover with a piece of parchment or wax paper cut to fit the pan. Bake for 25 minutes.
4. Meanwhile, add marinade to juices in skillet and simmer over low heat until reduced and thickened, about 15 minutes. Add a little freshly ground pepper, if you like. Pass the sauce separately.

Yield: 6 servings

Nutritive values per 1-breast serving:	CAL	CHO (gm)	PRO (gm)	FAT (gm)
	195	3	21	11

Food exchanges per 1-breast serving: 3 lean MEAT

BBQ Chicken

This flexible recipe gives you a barbecue flavor whether you use your outdoor grill, your broiler, or your range.

  1 medium onion, chopped
  1 tablespoon olive or peanut oil
1¼ cups tomato sauce
  1 tablespoon Worcestershire sauce
  1 tablespoon cider vinegar
  1 small bay leaf
  ¼ teaspoon dry mustard
  ¼ teaspoon ground cumin
  ¼ teaspoon hot pepper sauce
  ⅛ teaspoon freshly ground pepper
  1 3-pound broiler-fryer, cut into serving-size
    pieces and skinned

1. Sauté onion in oil in medium saucepan until tender. Stir in remaining ingredients except chicken and simmer 15 minutes. Remove bay leaf and discard.
2. Pour sauce over chicken in shallow baking dish. Cover and refrigerate for at least 4 hours, turning occasionally.
3. Grill chicken on barbecue or broil on foil-lined broiler pan 7 inches from heat. Cook 7–8 minutes on first side and 5 minutes after turning, until done. Baste often with marinade. A third cooking method: put chicken in large skillet, cover, and cook over low heat for 30 minutes. Uncover, turn chicken, and cook for another 15 minutes, until tender.

Yield: 6 servings

Nutritive values per serving:	CAL	CHO (gm)	PRO (gm)	FAT (gm)
	152	4	16	8

Food exchanges per serving: 2 lean MEAT, 1 VEGETABLE, ½ FAT

Oven-Fried Chicken

The best fried chicken I ever tasted was in Texas. It was so tender and tasty that I went to the kitchen and asked the cook for her secret. She told me she marinated the chicken overnight in vinegar. Here's a low-fat version of that tasty recipe.

1 cup white or cider vinegar
Skinned chicken pieces: 2 whole breasts (split), 2 legs and thighs
2 eggs
1 cup chicken broth
1½ cups fresh whole grain bread crumbs (made in blender)
½ cup grated Parmesan cheese
2 tablespoons paprika

1. The night before serving, pour vinegar over chicken. Turn to coat and cover. Refrigerate.
2. One hour before dinner, preheat oven to 325°F. Combine eggs and chicken broth in one shallow dish. Combine bread crumbs, cheese, and paprika in another. Dip each piece of chicken in egg, then crumbs. Bake in shallow baking dish for approximately 45 minutes.

Variation

Substitute 3 tablespoons sesame seeds for cheese. (The cheese and sesame seeds are approximately the same in calories and nutritional breakdown, so there is no real difference in exchanges in this variation.)

Yield: 6 servings (1 breast or 1 leg and thigh per serving)

Nutritive values per serving:

CAL	CHO (gm)	PRO (gm)	FAT (gm)
347	30	29	12

Food exchanges per serving: 2 BREAD, 3½ lean MEAT, trace FAT

Peanut Butter Chicken

Serve with noodles or brown rice, steamed vegetables, and fresh pineapple or a lemon dessert like Lemon Snow (see index for recipe) to balance the peanut butter flavor.

3 cloves garlic, minced
1 medium onion, sliced
1 28-ounce can tomatoes, whirled in blender
¾ cup white wine
3 pounds chicken pieces, skinned
¼ cup natural peanut butter

1. Combine all ingredients except peanut butter in large skillet and simmer, covered, 45 minutes.
2. Remove chicken. Add peanut butter. Stir and heat. Pour sauce over chicken and serve.

Yield: 6 servings

Nutritive values per serving:	CAL	CHO (gm)	PRO (gm)	FAT (gm)
	203	8	18	11

Food exchanges per serving: 2 lean MEAT, 1½ VEGETABLE, 1 FAT

Chicken Pizzaiola

I had this in the home of Cynthia Wadnola, a JDF volunteer, and it was terrific. I've reduced the fat used, but the recipe is just as good. More veggies!

½ cup each chopped: sweet red peppers,
  celery, carrots, green peppers, zucchini,
  and yellow squash
2 cloves garlic, minced
1 medium onion, sliced
½ cup sliced fresh mushrooms
½ cup sliced pitted black olives
½ cup white wine
4 cups tomato sauce
½ teaspoon basil leaves
½ teaspoon oregano leaves
¼ cup minced fresh parsley
6 chicken breast halves, skinned and boned
2 eggs, beaten
1 cup whole grain bread crumbs (made in
  blender)
1 tablespoon olive oil
8 ounces part-skim mozzarella cheese, sliced
  in 6 even slices

1. Simmer, covered, all vegetables, olives, wine, tomato sauce, and seasonings for 1 hour.
2. Flatten breasts with a mallet. Dip in egg and then bread crumbs. Sauté in olive oil until golden on both sides. Transfer to baking dish. Preheat oven to 325°F.
3. Spoon sauce over chicken. Cover and bake for 15 minutes.
4. Uncover and place 1 slice of cheese on each breast. Spoon some sauce over the cheese and place under broiler for a few minutes, until cheese melts.

Yield: 6 servings

Nutritive values per serving:		CHO (gm)	PRO (gm)	FAT (gm)
	CAL			
	510	37	41	21

Food exchanges per serving: 1½ BREAD, 4½ lean MEAT, 3 VEGETABLE, 1½ FAT

Chicken Cordon Bleu

Serve lemon wedges to squeeze over this dish.

8 chicken breast halves, skinned and boned
8 teaspoons chopped fresh parsley
4 ounces part-skim mozzarella cheese, cut into 8 thin slices
4 ounces boiled ham, cut into 4 thin slices and halved
1 tablespoon diet mayonnaise
1 tablespoon warm water
¼ cup whole grain bread crumbs (made in blender)

1. Preheat oven to 325°F.
2. Pound breasts until they are thin. Sprinkle with parsley. Top each with a slice of cheese, then a half-slice of ham. Roll up tightly.
3. Stir together mayonnaise and water in shallow dish. Roll each chicken fillet in the mayonnaise mixture, then in the bread crumbs. Arrange the chicken rolls, seam side down, in a single layer on a nonstick or foil-lined baking sheet. Bake 20–25 minutes or until browned, cooked through, and cheese is melted.

Yield: 8 servings

Nutritive values per serving:		CHO (gm)	PRO (gm)	FAT (gm)
	CAL			
	258	4	29	14

Food exchanges per serving: ⅓ BREAD, 4 lean MEAT, ½ FAT

Brunswick Stew

This is a one-pot meal that makes for easy clean-up. Lima beans are a traditional ingredient, but peas are a good substitute for the kid who says, "Limas? Ugh!" If you don't have homemade stock handy, use the low-sodium canned.

1 roasting chicken (about 4–5 pounds), cut into serving pieces and skinned
2 cups water
4 cups homemade chicken stock
2 cups chopped celery
2 medium onions, chopped
1 cup chopped green pepper
1 clove garlic, minced
¼ cup chopped fresh parsley
1 teaspoon dried thyme
3 tablespoons Worcestershire sauce
1 teaspoon hot pepper sauce
1 28-ounce can crushed tomatoes *or* 4 large tomatoes, peeled and chopped
½ teaspoon freshly ground pepper
1 16-ounce bag frozen corn
1 10-ounce package frozen lima beans *or* peas

1. In Dutch oven, combine chicken, water, stock, celery, onions, green pepper, garlic, parsley, thyme, Worcestershire sauce, hot pepper sauce, tomatoes, and pepper. Bring to a boil. Reduce heat, cover, and simmer 1 hour.
2. Remove chicken and cool. Remove meat from bones and return to Dutch oven; discard bones. Add corn and lima beans or peas. Simmer 30 minutes.

Yield: 8 approximately 2-cup servings

Nutritive values per approximate 2-cup serving:	CAL	CHO (gm)	PRO (gm)	FAT (gm)
	258	30	21	6

Food exchanges per approximate
2-cup serving: 2 BREAD, 2½ lean MEAT

TURKEY

Turkey Loaf

Try this instead of meat loaf.

  2 pounds ground turkey
  1 cup shredded carrots
  ½ cup quick (not instant) oats
  ½ cup chopped celery
  ¼ cup chopped onion
  ¼ cup minced fresh parsley
  1 egg
  ¼ cup water
  ½ teaspoon each: sage, thyme, marjoram, and
    oregano leaves
  1 teaspoon Worcestershire sauce
  ½ teaspoon freshly ground pepper
  ¼ cup catsup
  ¾ teaspoon dry mustard

1. Preheat oven to 350°F.
2. In a medium bowl, combine turkey, carrots, oats, celery, onion, parsley, egg, water, herbs, Worcestershire sauce, and pepper. Press into a 9- by 5-inch loaf pan.
3. In a small bowl, combine catsup and mustard. Spoon over meat loaf. Bake 45 minutes. Cut into 8 equal slices.

Yield: 8 servings

	CAL	CHO (gm)	PRO (gm)	FAT (gm)
Nutritive values per serving:	200	8	24	8

Food exchanges per serving: 3 lean MEAT, 1½ VEGETABLE

Roast Stuffed Turkey

Roast turkey is a low-fat protein source that's easy to prepare, and I roast a whole turkey about once a month. I use the leftovers for sandwiches, soup, and Turkey Chili (see index for recipe). Also, be sure to save the turkey carcass for stock. Cover it with water and simmer for several hours. Add a few chopped carrots, celery stalks, an onion or two, and ½ lemon, sliced. Strain. Refrigerate until fat solidifies, then remove fat and use stock for soup or other recipes. Use it in any recipe that calls for chicken broth. My favorite stuffing recipe follows this one. Concerning the cooking time, it's usually recommended that you cook a stuffed turkey 15–20 minutes per pound. I have found that cooking the turkey completely covered, as I describe here, cuts the cooking time for a 12-pound turkey by 45 minutes to 1 hour. I've recommended 3–3½ hours, but it may be done before 3 hours. Start checking the thermometer after 2½ hours.

> 1   12-pound turkey, fresh or defrosted
>   Freshly ground black pepper to taste
> 12   cups Stuffing for Turkey (recipe follows)
> 1   cup white wine
>   Paprika

1. Preheat oven to 325°F.
2. Wash the bird and dry it with paper towels. Sprinkle the cavity with pepper.
3. Spoon in the stuffing (do not pack tightly), leaving a little space at the end for expansion. If the neck skin is available, stuff that, too. Sew up the open ends (try dental floss instead of thread) or close with skewers and cord. (That's the traditional way to do it. I don't, and I've never had stuffing fall out of a turkey.)
4. Place the turkey breast side up on a rack in a roasting pan big enough to hold it without squeezing it. Pour wine over, sprinkle with paprika, and cover with foil or

pan cover if it fits. Roast the bird for approximately 3–
$3\frac{1}{2}$ hours (or until a thermometer inserted in the bird's
thigh registers 180–185°F), removing the cover and
basting the turkey with the pan juices several times
during the last 30–60 minutes. For an unstuffed turkey, reduce the roasting time by about 30 minutes.

5. To serve, transfer the stuffing to a separate bowl before
carving the turkey. Serve the turkey without the skin.
Turkey skin is much less fatty than chicken but still
would add 90 calories and 2 FAT exchanges per ounce.

Yield: 12 servings

Nutritive values per 5-ounce serving:	CAL	CHO (gm)	PRO (gm)	FAT (gm)
	275	0	35	15

Food exchanges per 5-ounce
serving: 5 lean MEAT

Stuffing for Turkey

I make the cornbread fresh or use half of a recipe that's left over from breakfast. If you're not that ambitious, use the whole wheat bread. Lots of fiber and sneaky vegetables in this one!

> 1 recipe Gloria's Cornbread (see index for recipe) *or* 1 1-pound loaf whole wheat bread *or* ½ recipe Gloria's Cornbread and ½ loaf whole wheat bread
> ¼ cup minced fresh parsley
> 2 medium apples, cored, unpeeled, and chopped
> 2 medium onions, chopped
> 3 stalks celery, diced
> 3 medium carrots, grated
> ¼ head green cabbage, chopped
> 1 cup chicken broth
> 1 teaspoon basil leaves
> 2 teaspoons sage leaves
> Freshly ground pepper

1. Crumble the bread or cornbread by hand or cut it into cubes.
2. Sauté the apple and the vegetables with chicken broth for 10 minutes over medium heat.
3. Combine all ingredients in a large bowl. (You'll probably have more stuffing than the turkey can hold. Put it into a 1-quart casserole, sprinkle with ¼ cup skim milk, cover, and bake at 325°F for 40–45 minutes.)

Yield: 12 servings

Nutritive values with Whole Wheat Bread, per serving:	CAL	CHO (gm)	PRO (gm)	FAT (gm)
	116	25	4	0

Food exchanges with Whole Wheat Bread, per serving: 1⅔ BREAD

Nutritive values with ½ bread and
½ cornbread, per serving:

CAL	CHO (gm)	PRO (gm)	FAT (gm)
141	27	5	1

Food exchanges with ½ bread and
½ cornbread, per serving:

2 BREAD, trace FAT

Nutritive values with cornbread,
per serving:

CAL	CHO (gm)	PRO (gm)	FAT (gm)
167	29	6	3

Food exchanges with cornbread,
per serving:

2 BREAD, ½ FAT

Turkey Burgers

Try these as a low-fat alternative to hamburgers.

    1 pound ground turkey
    ½ cup whole grain bread crumbs (made in
      blender from 2 slices bread)
    2 tablespoons finely chopped onion
    2 tablespoons fresh lemon juice
    1 teaspoon Worcestershire sauce
    ½ teaspoon paprika
      Freshly ground black pepper to taste

1. Combine all ingredients and shape the mixture into 6
   patties.
2. Fry, broil, or grill the burgers until they are done,
   about 5 minutes a side.

Yield: 6 servings

Nutritive values per serving:

CAL	CHO (gm)	PRO (gm)	FAT (gm)
138	6	15	6

Food exchanges per serving:

⅓ BREAD, 2 lean MEAT

Turkey Tetrazzini

Here's one good way to use leftover turkey.

- ¼ pound mushrooms, sliced
- 1 tablespoon diet margarine
- 2 tablespoons unbleached white flour
- ½ teaspoon salt
- ½ teaspoon freshly ground pepper
- ⅛ teaspoon cayenne pepper
- 2 cups skim milk
- 1 teaspoon Worcestershire sauce
- ½ cup shredded Swiss or Gruyère cheese
- ⅓ cup sliced green onions
- 2 cups cooked turkey or chicken (about ½ pound), cut into small cubes
- ½ pound spaghetti, cooked al dente and drained
- ¼ cup grated Parmesan cheese

1. Preheat oven to 350°F.
2. In a large saucepan over medium heat, sauté the mushrooms in the margarine, stirring them often, until they are just tender.
3. Stir in the flour, salt, pepper, and cayenne. Gradually add the milk, stirring constantly. Add the Worcestershire sauce and simmer the sauce, stirring, until it has thickened.
4. Add the cheese and green onions to the sauce and mix well. Add half the sauce to the turkey and half to the spaghetti.
5. Place the spaghetti in the bottom of a greased 2-quart baking dish. Make a well in the center and pour in the turkey. Sprinkle with Parmesan cheese.
6. Bake for 20 minutes, until heated through.

Yield: 6 1-cup servings

Nutritive values per 1-cup serving:	CAL	CHO (gm)	PRO (gm)	FAT (gm)
	287	35	21	7

Food exchanges per 1-cup serving:

2½ BREAD, 2 lean MEAT, trace FAT

FISH

The secret to properly cooked fish is timing. Overcooking toughens and dries it. The rule the professionals use is called the "10-minute rule": cook 10 minutes per inch of thickness. As fish cooks, it turns from translucent to opaque, like egg whites. To test if it's done, insert a fork at its thickest point, and if the fish looks opaque, it's ready. If it flakes easily, you've probably overcooked it. Fish that is baked, simmered, or enclosed in foil takes longer than fish that's broiled, fried, or poached. Use a 15-minute rule in that case.

Seafood Stew

This is actually a very easy bouillabaisse.

> 1 cup chopped onion
> 1 clove garlic, minced
> 2 cups chopped fresh tomatoes
> 2 10½-ounce cans condensed beef broth (preferably low-sodium)
> ½ cup cream sherry
> 4 lemon slices
> 3 whole allspice
> 1 bay leaf
> 1 pound skinned fish fillets
> 1 pound shrimp, deveined
> 1 dozen clams *or* 1 10-ounce can chopped clams, undrained
> ¼ cup grated Parmesan cheese

1. Simmer onion, garlic, tomatoes, beef broth, sherry, lemon slices, and seasonings, uncovered, for 30 minutes.
2. Cut fish fillets into large chunks. Add fish, shrimp, and clams to pot. Simmer 15–20 minutes or until clams open. Top with grated Parmesan cheese. Serve with salad and garlic bread.

Yield: 6 1½-cup servings

Nutritive values per 1½-cup serving:	CAL	CHO (gm)	PRO (gm)	FAT (gm)
	199	5	38	3

Food exchanges per 1½-cup
serving: 5½ lean MEAT, 1 VEGETABLE

Oven "French-Fried" Scallops

Many kids, including my own, love these easy and tasty scallops.

1 pound fresh or frozen and defrosted scallops
½ cup low-calorie Italian dressing
½ cup fresh whole grain bread crumbs (make in blender or food processor from 2 slices bread)
Paprika
Lemon slices

1. Preheat oven to 450°F.
2. Drain scallops and pat dry with a paper towel. Dip in dressing, then roll in bread crumbs. Sprinkle with paprika. For best results, refrigerate and allow to dry before baking.
3. Spread scallops in single layer in nonstick baking pan or cookie sheet. Bake 10 minutes per inch of thickness. Serve with lemon wedges.

Yield: 4 3-ounce servings

Nutritive values per 3-ounce serving:	CAL	CHO (gm)	PRO (gm)	FAT (gm)
	155	10	22	3

Food exchanges per 3-ounce
serving: ⅔ BREAD, 3 lean MEAT

Saucy Scallops

1½ cups water
1 cup dry white wine
¼ teaspoon salt
2 tablespoons minced onion
Dash freshly ground pepper
1 pound fresh bay or sea scallops
1 cup sliced fresh mushrooms
2 tablespoons diet margarine
2 tablespoons all-purpose flour
1 cup skim milk
¼ teaspoon freshly ground white pepper
½ cup shredded Swiss cheese
1 teaspoon Dijon mustard
2 tablespoons chopped fresh parsley
2 tablespoons minced fresh dill *or* 2
   teaspoons dried dillweed

1. Preheat oven to 375°F.
2. Combine first 5 ingredients in a medium saucepan; cover and simmer 5 minutes. Stir scallops and mushrooms into liquid mixture; cover and simmer 5 minutes.
3. Remove scallops and mushrooms from saucepan with a slotted spoon, reserving liquid in pan; set scallops and mushrooms aside. Bring liquid to a boil and cook, uncovered, 10 minutes or until liquid is reduced to about 1 cup.
4. Melt margarine in a heavy saucepan over low heat; add flour and cook 1 minute, stirring constantly (mixture will be dry). Gradually add 1 cup reduced liquid and milk to flour mixture; cook over medium heat, stirring constantly with a wire whisk, until thickened and bubbly. Add white pepper, cheese, mustard, parsley, and dill, stirring until cheese is melted.
5. Spoon scallops, mushrooms, and sauce into 1-quart casserole and brown under broiler for 3–4 minutes or until sauce turns golden brown and begins to bubble.

Yield: 4 1-cup servings

Nutritive values per 1-cup serving:	CAL	CHO (gm)	PRO (gm)	FAT (gm)
	228	9	30	8

Food exchanges per 1-cup serving: ½ BREAD, 4 lean MEAT

Foiled Fish Fillets

Here's an easy recipe for fish from Lanna Saunders, a wonderful actress and a very good cook.

> 1⅓ pounds red snapper fillets
> 4 small pieces peeled fresh gingerroot
> 4 teaspoons soy sauce
> 4 shallots, minced, or green onions, chopped

1. Preheat oven to 400°F.
2. Cut or divide fish into 4 equal portions. Place each on a square of heavy-duty aluminum foil. Top each with a slice of ginger, 1 teaspoon soy sauce, and 1 shallot or green onion.
3. Seal foil like an envelope. Bake for 10–12 minutes.

Variations
1. Use sole or other firm white fish and to each portion add 1 tablespoon fresh lemon juice and 1 tablespoon minced fresh parsley with green onion; omit ginger and soy sauce.
2. Use salmon fillets with 2 tablespoons vermouth; ¼ teaspoon dill; ½ clove garlic, minced; 1 green onion; and 1 new potato, cut into small pieces, on each. (For this variation, add 1 BREAD and 70 calories.)

Yield: 4 servings

Nutritive values per serving:	CAL	CHO (gm)	PRO (gm)	FAT (gm)
	185	2	33	5

Food exchanges per serving: 4½ lean MEAT

Oven Fish Fillets

1 8-ounce carton nonfat yogurt
¼ cup grated Parmesan cheese
2 tablespoons minced fresh parsley
½ onion, minced
3 tablespoons fresh lemon juice
1 clove garlic, minced
1 pound flounder or other fish fillets

1. Preheat oven to 375°F.
2. Combine first 6 ingredients in blender or food processor. Whirl just until smooth. Place fish in baking dish; spread sauce evenly over fillets.
3. Bake for 12–15 minutes. Fish should separate easily when a fork is inserted in the middle.

Yield: 4 3-ounce servings

Nutritive values per 3-ounce serving:	CAL	CHO (gm)	PRO (gm)	FAT (gm)
	152	4	25	4

Food exchanges per 3-ounce serving: ⅓ MILK, 3 lean MEAT

Salmon Croquettes

A lady named Mercedes Cornell who worked for me used to make these, and the boys loved them and still do.

1 7¾-ounce can salmon, drained and flaked
¼ cup bread crumbs (made in blender or food processor from 1 slice whole grain bread)
2 eggs, slightly beaten
2 tablespoons fresh lemon juice
¼ teaspoon freshly ground pepper
1 teaspoon dried dillweed *or* 1 tablespoon minced fresh dill
   Olive oil
½ cup finely chopped celery
⅓ cup finely chopped green onions
   Mustard Sauce (recipe follows)

1. Combine first 6 ingredients; set aside.
2. Coat a large nonstick skillet with 1 teaspoon olive oil; place over medium heat until hot. Add celery and green onions; sauté until tender. Add to salmon mixture; mix well.
3. Coat skillet again with ½ teaspoon olive oil; place over medium-high heat until hot. For each salmon cake, spoon about ¼ cup mixture onto skillet; shape into patty with a spatula. Cook about 2 minutes or until browned on each side. Serve immediately with Mustard Sauce (recipe follows).

Yield: 4 servings (2 croquettes each)

Nutritive values per 2-croquette serving:	CAL	CHO (gm)	PRO (gm)	FAT (gm)
	208	12	22	8

Food exchanges per 2-croquette serving: 1 BREAD, 3 lean MEAT

Mustard Sauce

  2 tablespoons diet margarine
1½ tablespoons unbleached white flour
  1 cup skim milk
  1 teaspoon Dijon mustard
  1 tablespoon fresh lemon juice
  ¼ teaspoon salt

1. Melt margarine over low heat; add flour, stirring until smooth. Cook 1 minute, stirring constantly.
2. Gradually add milk; cook over medium heat, stirring constantly, until thickened and bubbly. Remove from heat; stir in mustard, lemon juice, and salt.

Yield: 1 cup

Nutritive values per 2-tablespoon serving:	CAL	CHO (gm)	PRO (gm)	FAT (gm)
	30	2	11	2

Food exchanges per 2-tablespoon serving: ½ FAT

MEAT DISHES

Meat is an excellent source of protein and the B vitamins as well as iron. Use lean choices with all visible fat trimmed. Serve meat with lots of side dishes so that the meat doesn't become the focal point of the meal.

BEEF

Lean Pastichio

This is a Greek dish of beef and pasta with a low-fat cheese sauce. Feta cheese is very strong and interesting in flavor, but some children may find it too strong. It can also be very salty. Try soaking it in cold water for 20 minutes, then draining, to rid it of some salt.

- ¾ pound lean ground round
- ½ cup chopped onion
- 1 cup uncooked elbow macaroni (whole wheat, if possible)
- 1 8-ounce can low-sodium tomato sauce
- 2 tablespoons grated Parmesan cheese
- 1 medium zucchini, diced
- ½ teaspoon thyme leaves
- ¼ teaspoon ground cinnamon
- ½ cup skim milk
- 3 tablespoons unbleached white flour
- ¼ teaspoon white pepper
- 1 cup skim milk
- ¼ cup plus 2 tablespoons grated Parmesan cheese
- ½ cup crumbled feta cheese (optional)
- 2 eggs, beaten
  Ground cinnamon

1. Preheat oven to 375°F.
2. Cook meat and onion in a large nonstick skillet over

medium-high heat until meat is browned; drain meat in a colander and pat dry with paper towels.

3. Cook macaroni according to package directions, omitting salt. Combine meat mixture, macaroni, and next 5 ingredients; spread in bottom of a 10- by 6- by 2-inch baking dish.

4. Combine ½ cup milk, flour, and pepper in a jar; cover tightly and shake vigorously to blend. Pour into a small saucepan and stir in 1 cup milk. Cook over medium heat, stirring constantly, until mixture is thickened and bubbly. Remove from heat and stir in ¼ cup plus 2 tablespoons Parmesan cheese and feta cheese. Let cool to room temperature.

5. Stir eggs into thickened milk mixture; pour evenly over meat mixture. Sprinkle lightly with cinnamon. Bake for 30–35 minutes or until knife inserted near center comes out clean. Let stand 10 minutes before serving. Divide into 6 equal portions.

Yield: 6 approximately 1-cup servings

Nutritive values without feta, per approximately 1-cup serving:	CAL	CHO (gm)	PRO (gm)	FAT (gm)
	263	21	20	11

Food exchanges without feta, per approximately 1-cup serving:

1 BREAD, 2 medium-fat MEAT 1 VEGETABLE

Nutritive values with feta, per approximately 1-cup serving:	CAL	CHO (gm)	PRO (gm)	FAT (gm)
	289	21	22	13

Food exchanges with feta, per approximately 1-cup serving:

1 BREAD, 2½ medium-fat MEAT, 1 VEGETABLE

Beef and Tomato Stir-Fry

My boys first had this at their grandma's and cleaned their plates.

1 pound lean top round steak, sliced thin across the grain
1 tablespoon cornstarch
2 tablespoons soy sauce (preferably reduced-sodium)
1 tablespoon peeled and minced fresh gingerroot
1 clove garlic, minced
1 teaspoon dark sesame oil
2 green onions, sliced thin
1 medium red pepper, cut into 1-inch chunks
1 medium green pepper, cut into 1-inch chunks
1 tablespoon water
1 medium zucchini, cut into ¼-inch slices
3 large tomatoes, seeded and cut into wedges
1 cup tomato juice
2 teaspoons Worcestershire sauce
3 cups hot, cooked rice

1. Place beef in a large, shallow glass baking dish. In small bowl, combine cornstarch, soy sauce, ginger, and garlic. Pour over beef; cover and marinate several hours or overnight.
2. In large skillet, heat oil. Stir-fry meat in batches until browned. Remove meat and reserve. Add green onion, red and green pepper, and 1 tablespoon water to skillet; cover and cook 1 minute. Add zucchini; cover and cook 1 minute.
3. Add tomatoes and meat to skillet.
4. Add tomato juice and Worcestershire sauce to skillet; stir to combine well. Cook until thickened. Serve over rice.

Yield: 4 servings (1¼ cups plus ¾ cup rice each)

	CAL	CHO (gm)	PRO (gm)	FAT (gm)
Nutritive values per serving (1¼ cups plus ¾ cup rice):	350	36	29	10

Food exchanges per serving
(1¼ cups plus ¾ cup rice): ½ BREAD, 3 lean MEAT, 3 VEGETABLE

Oriental Flank Steak

I serve this with Chinese Vegetables (see index for recipe) and Korean rice, and it's one of our favorite meals.

- 2 tablespoons dark sesame oil
- 3 cloves garlic, minced
- ¾ teaspoon ground ginger *or* 2 slices peeled fresh gingerroot, minced
- ½ cup low-sodium soy sauce *or* ¼ cup regular soy sauce and ¼ cup water
- ½ cup cream sherry
- 4 green onions, chopped
- 2 flank steaks (approximately 1¼ pounds each)

The night before serving, combine first 6 ingredients and pour over steaks in a shallow pan. Turn once or twice. The next day, broil steaks 6–7 minutes per side. (I use an indoor BBQ-type broiler.) Meanwhile, heat the marinade for 10–15 minutes. Slice the steaks thin across the grain, diagonally (à la London Broil) and pour marinade over to serve.

Yield: 8 4-ounce servings

	CAL	CHO (gm)	PRO (gm)	FAT (gm)
Nutritive values per 4-ounce serving:	250	0	28	15

Food exchanges per 4-ounce
serving: 4 lean MEAT, ½ FAT

Beef and Snow Peas

Chinese stir-fry dishes are great because they are made in one pan, have lots of vegetables, are low-fat, and cook quickly. See if you can get Korean rice. It has a round kernel and is slightly transparent. It's sometimes available in large supermarkets. Oyster sauce is available in Oriental markets and some supermarkets.

1　pound flank steak, semifrozen, cut into thin slices across grain
2　tablespoons cream sherry
2　tablespoons rice vinegar
2　tablespoons soy sauce (preferably reduced-sodium)
2　tablespoons cornstarch
2　teaspoons dark sesame oil
1　pound Chinese pea pods, stem ends cut off
¼　head green cabbage, chopped
¼　pound mushrooms, cleaned and sliced
1　teaspoon dark sesame oil
2　slices peeled fresh gingerroot, minced
1　clove garlic, minced
2　tablespoons broth or water
1　tablespoon oyster sauce

1. Marinate steak in sherry, vinegar, soy sauce, and cornstarch overnight in refrigerator.
2. Heat 2 teaspoons sesame oil in wok or large skillet until hot. Add pea pods, cabbage, and mushrooms. Stir-fry a few minutes. Remove vegetables and reserve.
3. Add 1 teaspoon sesame oil to wok and stir-fry ginger and garlic for 1 minute. Add steak to wok and stir-fry until the steak loses its pinkness. Add vegetables, broth, and oyster sauce. Cover and steam for 1 minute.

Yield: 6 1-cup servings

Nutritive values per 1-cup serving:	CAL	CHO (gm)	PRO (gm)	FAT (gm)
	164	7	16	8

Food exchanges per 1-cup
serving: 2 lean MEAT, 1½ VEGETABLE,
                                  ½ FAT

Pot Roast

I use a seven-bone, round-bone, or top round roast.

    1 3-pound beef pot roast, trimmed of visible
       fat
    1 lemon
    2 medium onions, sliced thin
    6 small carrots
    1 clove garlic, minced
    2 medium unpeeled potatoes, quartered
    1 teaspoon dry mustard
    1 teaspoon ground ginger
    1 teaspoon thyme leaves
    4 stalks celery, with leaves, chopped
    1 small green pepper, cut up
    2 cups tomato *or* vegetable juice

1. The night before serving, put roast in a glass casserole and squeeze lemon over it. Pierce with a fork, cover tightly, and refrigerate.
2. Preheat oven to 325°F about 3 hours before dinner.
3. Put roast in large casserole with a cover. Put onions, carrots, garlic, and potatoes around meat. Sprinkle mustard, ginger, and thyme over meat. Place celery and green pepper on top of meat.
4. Pour tomato or vegetable juice around meat. Cover and bake until fork-tender, about 3 hours.

Yield: 6 4½-ounce servings

Nutritive values per 4½-ounce serving:	CAL	CHO (gm)	PRO (gm)	FAT (gm)
	378	11	34	22

Food exchanges per 4½-ounce
serving: 1 BREAD, 4½ medium-fat
                                  MEAT

Vegetable and Meat Loaf

Using lean ground round instead of ground beef decreases the amount of fat and calories, especially when cooked in the manner described below. Use a baster to siphon off the liquefied fats and juices that collect in the pan during cooking. More fiber, less meat!

1½ pounds lean ground round
½ cup soft whole wheat bread crumbs (made in blender)
½ cup shredded carrots
¼ cup thinly sliced celery
½ onion, minced
¼ cup chopped green pepper
1 egg, slightly beaten
1 small bunch fresh spinach, cleaned, stemmed, and chopped (½ pound)
2 teaspoons Worcestershire sauce
½ teaspoon dry mustard
½ teaspoon freshly ground pepper
2 tablespoons minced fresh parsley
¼ cup tomato puree
1 16-ounce can whole tomatoes
1 teaspoon basil leaves

1. Preheat oven to 350°F.
2. Combine all ingredients except tomato puree, tomatoes, and basil. Shape into a loaf. Place in shallow baking dish. Pour puree over and bake for 1 hour or until done.
3. Whirl the tomatoes briefly in a blender or food processor. There should still be some small lumps of tomato. Add the basil. Transfer to a small saucepan and simmer, uncovered, for 10–15 minutes. Serve the sauce separately.
4. Lift meat loaf out of drippings with 2 large spatulas. Cut into 6 equal portions. They will be approximately ¾ cup in volume.

Yield: 6 servings

Nutritive values per serving:	CAL	CHO (gm)	PRO (gm)	FAT (gm)
	213	12	22	9

Food exchanges per serving: 3 lean MEAT, 1 VEGETABLE

Swiss Steak

1 2-pound round steak
3 tablespoons unbleached white flour
½ teaspoon salt
½ teaspoon freshly ground pepper
½ teaspoon paprika
1 tablespoon olive oil
1 medium onion, chopped
½ cup each chopped carrots, celery, and green pepper
¼ cup chopped fresh parsley
1 16-ounce can tomatoes with liquid
1 cup sliced fresh mushrooms
1 tablespoon cornstarch
¼ cup cold water

1. Trim fat and bone from meat and cut into 6 equal portions. Mix flour, salt, pepper, and paprika and sprinkle over both sides of the meat. Pound in with a mallet or the edge of a plate. Brown meat in oil in a large skillet.
2. Add onion, carrots, celery, green pepper, parsley, and tomatoes. Cover and simmer for 2 hours. Add mushrooms for the last 10 minutes.
3. Remove meat from pan and add the cornstarch that has been stirred into the water to the skillet. Cook over medium heat, stirring, until thickened. Serve sauce over meat portions.

Yield: 6 servings

Nutritive values per serving:	CAL	CHO (gm)	PRO (gm)	FAT (gm)
	302	13	31	14

Food exchanges per serving: ½ BREAD, 4 lean MEAT, 1 VEGETABLE, ½ FAT

Superb Oven Stew

This is my mother's recipe, but I added the carrots, potatoes, and peas. Try serving steamed broccoli and a salad to complete the meal.

 2 pounds lean beef, cut into 1-inch cubes
 ½ cup unbleached white flour
 2 tablespoons olive oil
 2 medium onions cut into ¼-inch slices
 3 cloves garlic, minced or pressed
 ¼ cup chopped fresh parsley
 ½ teaspoon thyme leaves
1½ cups beef stock (preferably low-sodium)
 1 cup beer
 6 carrots, cut into 1-inch chunks
 3 unpeeled medium potatoes, quartered
 1 cup frozen green peas
 1 tablespoon wine vinegar

1. Preheat oven to 325°F.
2. Coat meat with flour and brown in oil in heavy skillet.
3. Layer meat and onions in 2-quart casserole.
4. Sauté garlic in skillet. Add parsley, thyme, and beef stock. Scrape bottom of pan to loosen meat particles. Pour over meat in casserole. Pour beer over meat.
5. Cover casserole and bake for 1½ hours. Add carrots and potatoes and bake for 45 minutes more, covered. Add peas and wine vinegar, stir in, and bake, uncovered, for 10–15 minutes.

Yield: 6 1½-cup servings

Nutritive values per 1½-cup serving:	CAL	CHO (gm)	PRO (gm)	FAT (gm)
	352	29	32	12

Food exchanges per 1½-cup serving:		
	2 BREAD, 4 lean MEAT	

VEAL

Veal Scaloppine

1 pound ¼-inch-thick veal cutlets
3 tablespoons unbleached white flour
½ teaspoon salt
½ teaspoon freshly ground pepper
1 tablespoon olive oil
⅔ cup Chablis or other dry white wine
2 teaspoons Dijon mustard
¼ cup fresh lemon juice
Lemon zest twists (optional)

1. Trim excess fat from veal; place veal on a sheet of wax paper. Flatten to ⅛-inch thickness, using a meat mallet or rolling pin; cut into 2-inch pieces. Combine flour, salt, and pepper; dredge veal in flour mixture.
2. Add oil to a large skillet and place over medium-high heat until hot. Add veal and cook 1 minute on each side or until lightly browned. Remove veal from skillet and set aside.
3. Pour wine, mustard, and lemon juice into skillet; bring to a boil. Return veal to skillet, turning to coat with sauce; reduce heat, and simmer 1–2 minutes or until sauce is slightly thickened and veal is thoroughly heated. Garnish with lemon twists, if desired. Divide into 4 equal portions.

Yield: 4 servings

Nutritive values per serving:	CAL	CHO (gm)	PRO (gm)	FAT (gm)
	220	6	22	12

Food exchanges per serving: ⅓ BREAD, 3 lean MEAT, ½ FAT

Osso Buco

This classic dish is also known as Baked Marrow Bones or Braised Veal Shinbones. Serve with noodles and steamed vegetables and Carrot-Acorn Squash (see index).

    1 tablespoon extra-virgin olive oil
    4 pounds veal shanks (or shinbones), cut
      into 2-inch chunks and trimmed of fat
    2 onions, chopped
    1 clove garlic, minced
    2 bay leaves
    1 teaspoon rosemary leaves
    ½ teaspoon freshly ground pepper
    1 cup dry white wine vinegar
    1 carrot, grated
    1 celery stalk, minced
    2 tablespoons red wine
    1 tablespoon grated lemon zest
    ¼ cup chopped fresh parsley
    2 cups chopped fresh tomatoes
    2 tablespoons tomato paste
    ½ cup water or stock

1. Preheat oven to 325°F.
2. Using a Dutch oven, heat olive oil over medium-high heat and sear the cut sides of the veal shanks. Add the onions, garlic, bay leaves, rosemary, pepper, and white wine vinegar. Cover and reduce heat to low. Simmer for 5 minutes.
3. Add the carrot, celery, red wine, lemon zest, parsley, and tomatoes. Stir the tomato paste into the water or stock and add to the veal. Mix well.
4. Transfer covered Dutch oven to oven and bake for 1½–2 hours, until tender. Remove the veal and place on serving platter. Discard the bay leaves.

5. Over medium-high heat, cook the remaining sauce for several minutes to reduce the volume and to thicken. Pour the sauce over the shanks and serve.

Yield: 8 1-cup servings

Nutritive values per 1-cup serving:	CAL	CHO (gm)	PRO (gm)	FAT (gm)
	189	4	23	9

Food exchanges per 1-cup serving: 3 lean MEAT, 1 VEGETABLE

Veal Chops with Raspberry Vinegar

This is a gourmet recipe that I included mainly for special occasions, because veal chops can be expensive for a family meal.

> 4 loin veal chops (¾–1 inch thick)
> ½ teaspoon salt
> ½ teaspoon freshly ground pepper
> 1 tablespoon unsalted butter
> 4 whole garlic cloves, unpeeled
> 2 bay leaves
> ½ teaspoon thyme leaves
> 1 tablespoon raspberry vinegar
> 1 cup chicken broth
> 1 tablespoon arrowroot
> 1 tablespoon cold water

1. Sprinkle chops with salt and pepper. Heat butter in large skillet and add chops. Brown on both sides, turning once, about 5 minutes on each side. Add garlic, bay leaves, and thyme and cook 3 minutes.
2. Pour the vinegar around the chops and turn heat to high for a few seconds, turning chops to coat both sides. Turn heat down to simmer, adding ½ cup of broth, and cook, covered tightly, for 20 minutes. Turn the chops frequently and add a little more broth when necessary, saving some for last.
3. When done, remove garlic and bay leaves and place chops on a warm platter. Mix about a teaspoon of arrowroot with 1 tablespoon cold water. Add remaining broth to the skillet and slowly add arrowroot mixture until the sauce reaches desired thickness. (Use more or less arrowroot mixture according to your taste.) Spoon sauce over chops and serve at once.

Yield: 4 servings

Nutritive values per serving:

	CAL	CHO (gm)	PRO (gm)	FAT (gm)
	192	0	21	12

Food exchanges per serving: 3 lean MEAT, ½ FAT

LAMB

Greek Lamb Chops

Try serving this with a whole grain side dish like bulgur or kasha (buckwheat groats).

    4 ¾-inch-thick lean loin lamb chops,
       trimmed of fat
       Juice of 1 lemon
    1 tablespoon crushed dried mint leaves
   ⅛ teaspoon ground cinnamon
   ⅛ teaspoon ground nutmeg
       Fresh mint sprigs (optional)

Sprinkle chops with lemon juice and seasonings; puncture repeatedly with a fork. Wrap in plastic; refrigerate several hours. Broil or grill chops, turning once, until brown and crisp outside but still pink in the middle or until done as desired. Garnish with fresh mint sprigs, if desired.

Yield: 4 servings

Nutritive values per serving:

	CAL	CHO (gm)	PRO (gm)	FAT (gm)
	165	0	21	9

Food exchanges per serving: 3 lean MEAT

Lovely Lamb Stew

This is a low-calorie main dish from the Days of Our Lives Celebrity Cookbook, *contributed by Kaye Stevens, and published by Gloria Loring, 1981.*

1 teaspoon oil
2 pounds stewing lamb, cut into 2-inch cubes
½ cup unbleached white flour
1 teaspoon freshly ground pepper
2 cloves garlic, minced
2 teaspoons celery seeds
3 carrots, quartered
6 small white onions, halved
¼ cup minced fresh parsley
2 teaspoons Worcestershire sauce
3 cups tomato juice

Heat heavy, deep pan, greased lightly with oil. Dip lamb in flour. Brown well. Add all remaining ingredients. Cover and simmer until fork-tender, 1½–2 hours.

Yield: 6 1¼-cup servings

Nutritive values per 1¼-cup serving:	CAL	CHO (gm)	PRO (gm)	FAT (gm)
	293	14	30	13

Food exchanges per 1¼-cup serving: 1 BREAD, 4 lean MEAT

Baked Lamb Chops

4 ½-inch-thick loin lamb chops
1 tablespoon olive oil
½ cup unsweetened orange juice
2 tablespoons soy sauce (preferably low-sodium)
1 teaspoon ground ginger
2 cloves garlic, minced
¼ teaspoon freshly ground pepper
2 small oranges, peeled and sectioned

1. Trim excess fat from chops. Lightly brown chops in hot oil and drain on paper towels.
2. Place chops in a shallow baking dish. Combine orange juice, soy sauce, ginger, garlic, and pepper; pour marinade over chops. Cover with foil and refrigerate for 2 hours, turning once.
3. Remove from refrigerator, but do not uncover. Bake at 350°F for 45–55 minutes or until chops are tender. Place orange sections on chops, cover, and bake for 10 minutes more. Or grill the chops, reserving the marinade. In that case, heat the marinade and pass separately.

Yield: 4 servings

Nutritive values per serving:	CAL	CHO (gm)	PRO (gm)	FAT (gm)
	224	8	21	11

Food exchanges per serving: 1 FRUIT, 3 lean MEAT, ½ FAT

PORK

Orange Pork Chops with Rice

A delicious, almost one-dish meal. Serve with Broccoli Parmesan and Fruit Spiced Carrots (see index for recipes).

    4   ¾-inch-thick pork chops
    1   teaspoon olive oil
    1   cup long-grain brown rice
    1½ cups unsweetened orange juice
    1   small onion, chopped
    ½   teaspoon ground cinnamon
    ¼   teaspoon ground nutmeg
    ½   teaspoon freshly ground pepper
    1   large baking apple, unpeeled, cored, and
        cut crosswise into 4 slices
        Grated zest of ½ orange
    1   orange, peeled and cut into bite-size pieces
    2   tablespoons chopped fresh parsley

1. Trim excess fat from chops. Brown in oil in large skillet. Remove chops and wipe out any fat.
2. Place next 6 ingredients in skillet and bring to boil. Reduce heat and place chops over rice. Cover and cook for 20 minutes over low heat.
3. Place an apple slice on top of each chop. Cook 15 minutes longer, until all liquid is absorbed.
4. Remove chops and apple. Stir in orange zest, orange pieces, and parsley. Arrange rice mixture and chops topped with apples on a serving dish.

Yield: 4 servings

Nutritive values per serving:	CAL	CHO (gm)	PRO (gm)	FAT (gm)
	360	32	31	12

Food exchanges per serving: 1½ BREAD, 1 FRUIT, 4 lean MEAT

NOODLES, RICE, GRAINS, AND POTATOES
Noodle Kugel

This is another recipe from my mom that's been adjusted to be low-fat and low-sugar. My mother was born in Minnesota, of Norwegian descent, but I think she always secretly wanted to be a Jewish mother. She makes great noodle kugel and matzo ball soup! This is a good side dish for baked chicken; add a salad or steamed vegetables.

1 8-ounce package broad egg noodles
2 whole eggs
2 egg whites
8 packets artificial sweetener (equal to ⅓ cup sugar)
1 cup nonfat yogurt
1 cup low-fat cottage cheese
¾ cup evaporated skim milk
½ cup seedless raisins *or* ¼ cup raisins and ¼ cup diced dried apricots or currants
1 teaspoon vanilla extract
½ teaspoon ground cinnamon
¼ teaspoon ground nutmeg
1 teaspoon grated orange zest

1. Preheat oven to 350°F.
2. Cook noodles according to package directions. Drain.
3. In a large bowl, beat eggs, egg whites, and sweetener. Blend in all remaining ingredients. Add noodles and mix thoroughly.
4. Pour into a 2-quart baking dish and bake 1 hour.

Yield: 8 ¾-cup servings

Nutritive values per ¾-cup serving:	CAL	CHO (gm)	PRO (gm)	FAT (gm)
	200	30	13	3

Food exchanges per ¾-cup serving:

2 BREAD, 1 FRUIT, 1 lean MEAT

Red Beans and Rice

This dish is very good for many reasons. First of all, it's very high in fiber. Also, the combination of beans and rice makes this a complete protein. It can be served as a main dish with a salad and vegetable dish for a very nutritious meal.

¾ pound ham hocks
1 quart water
1 pound dried red beans
1½ cups chopped onion
1 cup chopped fresh parsley
1 cup chopped green pepper
½ cup chopped green onions
2 cloves garlic, pressed
1 8-ounce can tomato sauce
1 tablespoon Worcestershire sauce
1 teaspoon freshly ground pepper
½ teaspoon crushed red pepper
¼ teaspoon oregano leaves
¼ teaspoon thyme leaves
3 dashes hot red pepper sauce
5 cups hot cooked rice, long-grain brown or white

1. Wash ham hocks and place in a large saucepan. Add 1 quart water and bring to a boil. Cover, reduce heat, and simmer 30 minutes or until meat is tender. Remove ham hocks and discard. Strain broth and chill overnight or until fat rises to the surface and hardens. Remove the fat and discard; set broth aside.
2. Sort and wash beans; place in a Dutch oven. Cover with water and soak overnight.
3. Drain beans; combine beans and broth in Dutch oven. Cover and cook over low heat for 45 minutes. Add remaining ingredients except rice; cover and cook over low heat 2–2½ hours, stirring occasionally and adding additional water, if desired. Serve over rice.

Yield: 10 1-cup servings

Nutritive values per 1-cup serving:	CAL	CHO (gm)	PRO (gm)	FAT (gm)
	283	49	17	2

Food exchanges per 1-cup
serving: 3 BREAD, 1 lean MEAT,
1 VEGETABLE

Rice and Vegetable Casserole

Serve this with a green vegetable like steamed fresh green beans and baked chicken or fish. The combination of corn and rice makes this dish a complete protein.

4 small zucchini, chopped
6 green onions, chopped
1 cup fresh or frozen corn kernels
1 16-ounce can tomatoes, undrained and chopped
½ teaspoon freshly ground pepper
   Pinch each basil and thyme leaves
2 cups cooked long-grain brown rice

1. In a large skillet, place first 4 ingredients over medium heat and cook until they begin to boil. Reduce heat and simmer for 10 minutes, until tender and most of the liquid is gone.
2. Stir in the seasonings and rice. Heat for a few minutes.

Yield: 6 ¾-cup servings

Nutritive values per ¾-cup serving:	CAL	CHO (gm)	PRO (gm)	FAT (gm)
	104	22	4	0

Food exchanges per ¾-cup
serving: 1 BREAD, 1½ VEGETABLE

Bulgur Pilaf

Bulgur is cracked wheat. It is parboiled and then cracked into small pieces. It comes in three sizes: the largest for pilaf, the middle-sized for cereal, and the smallest for tabbouli, a Middle Eastern salad. It has a nutty flavor and is very dense, which means it has more calories than the same size serving of some other grains. At the same time, it has lots of fiber and is very filling.

For children used to instant rice (or "mush," as I call it), bulgur will be a shock. Try breaking them in slowly. Mix white rice and brown long-grain rice for a while. Then sneak in a little bulgur until your children get used to the brown kernels they need to chew!

     2 teaspoons diet margarine
     1 small onion, minced
     1 cup bulgur
     2 cups boiling homemade chicken stock or
        water
    ¼ teaspoon freshly ground pepper

1. Melt margarine in a medium saucepan. Sauté onion for 5 minutes. Add bulgur and cook for another 2 minutes.
2. Add stock and pepper. Stir. Cover and reduce heat to simmer for 15 minutes or until liquid is absorbed.

Yield: 6 ⅓-cup servings

Nutritive values per ⅓-cup serving:	CAL	CHO (gm)	PRO (gm)	FAT (gm)
	132	29	4	0

Food exchanges per ⅓-cup
serving: 2 BREAD

Oven "French Fries"

2 large potatoes
1 tablespoon olive oil
¼ teaspoon salt
¼ teaspoon freshly ground pepper
⅛ teaspoon paprika

1. Preheat oven to 350°F.
2. Cut potatoes into thin strips, leaving the skins on. In a medium bowl, sprinkle remaining ingredients over potatoes and toss thoroughly to coat.
3. Arrange potatoes on a nonstick baking sheet. Bake for 20 minutes. Using spatula, turn potatoes over. Bake 20 minutes longer, until browned and crisp.

Yield: 4 4-ounce servings

Nutritive values per 4-ounce serving:	CAL	CHO (gm)	PRO (gm)	FAT (gm)
	111	19	3	3

Food exchanges per 4-ounce serving: 1 BREAD, ½ FAT

Potato-Bean Patties

This recipe is reproduced completely from Jane Brody's Good Food Book.

"Even children who would otherwise never touch a bean devoured these soft croquettes, which have a crisp outer shell. They are excellent as a lunch or supper entree, accompanied by a green vegetable and salad. If you have precooked the beans, the patties can be prepared quickly. Adzuki (or aduki) beans are very small and kidney-red; they are widely available in natural food stores. The closest substitute would be small red beans. For added nutrients and flavor, use the potato water as part of the liquid for cooking the beans. The "batter" or patties can be fully prepared even a day ahead and refrigerated. Because the patties are soft, it is important to fry them with enough space between them so that they can be turned easily. They are easier to handle on a pancake griddle (preferably one with a nonstick surface) rather than a frying pan."

1 pound unpeeled potatoes, scrubbed and boiled in lightly salted water until tender
1 egg white
3 tablespoons skim milk
1 teaspoon butter or margarine
Freshly ground black pepper to taste
2 tablespoons minced fresh parsley
½ cup dried adzuki beans, soaked and cooked until tender but not mushy
½ cup grated Parmesan cheese
2–3 tablespoons vegetable oil

1. When the potatoes are cool enough to handle, peel and mash them with egg white, milk, butter or margarine, and pepper.
2. Stir in the parsley and fold in the cooked beans.
3. Form the mixture into 16 patties (about 2½ inches in diameter), coating each one on both sides with the grated cheese. Place them on a flat surface on a sheet

of wax paper, but do not let them touch.

4. In batches on an oiled griddle or in a skillet, fry the patties until they are browned on both sides, taking care when turning them not to mush them. Keep the cooked patties warm in the oven until serving time.

Yield: 8 servings (2 patties each)

Nutritive values per 2-patty serving:	CAL	CHO (gm)	PRO (gm)	FAT (gm)
	133	16	6	5

Food exchanges per 2-patty serving: 1 BREAD, 1 medium-fat MEAT

Potato Kugel

This is a recipe from my vegetarian friend, Wendy Iscov, who is also the mother of two boys.

> 5 medium potatoes, grated coarse
> 2 medium onions, chopped
> 2 eggs, beaten
> 2 cloves garlic, minced
> 1 teaspoon freshly ground pepper
> 1 teaspoon salt
> 3 tablespoons matzo meal

1. Preheat oven to 350°F.

2. Mix all ingredients completely. Pour into an oiled 9- by 13-inch baking dish. Bake for 1½ hours. Cut into 10 equal portions.

Yield: 10 ½-cup servings

Nutritive values per ½-cup serving:	CAL	CHO (gm)	PRO (gm)	FAT (gm)
	97	18	4	1

Food exchanges per ½-cup serving: 1 BREAD, trace FAT

Stuffed Yams

Yams have a good glycemic index rating. They raise blood sugar at a much slower rate and to a lower level than white potatoes.

> 2 medium yams (about 1½ pounds), scrubbed and baked
> ½ cup unsweetened, undrained crushed pineapple
> ¼ teaspoon ground cinnamon
> ¼ teaspoon ground nutmeg

1. Preheat oven to 400°F.
2. Cut each baked yam in half lengthwise. Scoop pulp into bowl, leaving shells intact.
3. Mash pulp with other ingredients. Spoon one-quarter of mixture into each shell. Bake about 15 minutes.

Yield: 4 ½-cup servings

Nutritive values per ½-cup serving:	CAL	CHO (gm)	PRO (gm)	FAT (gm)
	152	34	4	0

Food exchanges per ½-cup serving: 2 BREAD, ½ FRUIT

Puffed Sweet Potatoes

Like yams, sweet potatoes have good glycemic index ratings.

> 2 medium sweet potatoes, baked
> ¼ cup unsweetened orange juice
> ¼ teaspoon ground ginger
> ¼ teaspoon ground nutmeg
> 1 teaspoon grated orange zest
> 2 egg whites

1. Preheat oven to 350°F.
2. Peel sweet potatoes and mash pulp. Add juice, ginger, nutmeg, and grated zest.
3. Beat egg whites until stiff peaks form and fold them into sweet potato mixture. Spoon into a 1-quart non-stick baking dish and bake for 30 minutes.

Yield: 4 ½-cup servings

Nutritive values per ½-cup serving:	CAL	CHO (gm)	PRO (gm)	FAT (gm)
	116	31	5	0

Food exchanges per ½-cup serving: 2 BREAD

Sweet Potatoes and Bananas

I had this at my friend Bette Mazur's house. I took out the butter and sugar, and it's still great.

> 2 pounds sweet potatoes or yams, cooked and peeled
> 3 bananas, peeled and sliced
> ½ cup unsweetened orange juice
> 4 packets artificial sweetener (equal to 8 teaspoons sugar)
> ½ teaspoon ground cinnamon
> ¼ teaspoon ground nutmeg

1. Preheat oven to 375°F.
2. Slice potatoes. Toss bananas with ¼ cup orange juice.
3. In 2-quart baking dish, layer half the potatoes, then ⅔ of the sliced bananas. Mix the sweetener, cinnamon, and nutmeg and sprinkle half over the potatoes and bananas. Pour in any juice left over from tossing the bananas. Layer remaining potatoes; end with remaining bananas in the center. Pour remaining orange juice over and sprinkle with sweetener mixture.
4. Bake for 45 minutes, until bubbly.

Yield: 6 ⅔-cup servings

Nutritive values per ⅔-cup serving:	CAL	CHO (gm)	PRO (gm)	FAT (gm)
	112	25	3	0

Food exchanges per ⅔-cup
serving: 1 BREAD, 1 FRUIT

STARCHY VEGETABLES
Carrot-Acorn Squash

I could never get my younger son to eat acorn squash until I served it like this.

2 acorn squash (approximately 1½ pounds each)
2 cups cooked sliced carrots
1 tablespoon fresh lemon juice
¼ teaspoon each ground nutmeg and mace
1 tablespoon grated orange zest

1. Preheat oven to 350°F.
2. Cut squash in half lengthwise and remove seeds. Place cut side down on baking sheet and bake for 40–45 minutes, until tender.
3. Scoop out squash pulp. Put squash and carrots, juice, spices, and zest in blender or food processor. Whirl briefly. Don't let it turn to complete mush, or you lose the value of the fiber in the vegetables. Serve warm.

Variation
The quickest version of the recipe above is to make it without the carrots. Put the squash pulp in the blender or processor with ⅛ teaspoon nutmeg, ⅛ teaspoon mace, and 1 tablespoon orange zest.

Yield: 6 ¾-cup servings

Nutritive values per ¾-cup serving:	CAL	CHO (gm)	PRO (gm)	FAT (gm)
	92	20	3	0
Food exchanges per ¾-cup serving:	1 BREAD, 1 VEGETABLE			

Nutritive values Variation per serving:	CAL	CHO (gm)	PRO (gm)	FAT (gm)
	72	16	3	0
Food exchanges Variation per serving:	1 BREAD			

Corn Pudding

This is wonderful served with anything. It's even good for breakfast. The milk, eggs, and corn provide complete protein with some fiber. You can use diet margarine, but the taste will be a little different. I use the butter and balance it by serving it with other very low-fat dishes.

> 3 tablespoons butter, softened, or diet margarine
> 3 packets artificial sweetener (equal to 2 tablespoons sugar)
> 2 tablespoons unbleached white flour
> ½ teaspoon salt
> 2 whole eggs
> 3 egg whites
> 2 cups fresh corn kernels *or* 1 10-ounce bag frozen corn kernels
> 1⅓ cups evaporated skim milk
> ½ teaspoon ground cumin (optional)

1. Preheat oven to 325°F.
2. Blend butter, sweetener, flour, and salt.
3. Add eggs and egg whites and beat well. Stir in corn, milk, and cumin, if desired. Mix well. Pour into oiled 2-quart baking dish and bake for 45 minutes. Stir only once during baking. When done, it will be golden brown and of custard consistency. Knife inserted half-way between side and center should come out clean.

Yield: 6 ¾-cup servings

Nutritive values per ¾-cup serving:	CAL	CHO (gm)	PRO (gm)	FAT (gm)
	157	18	10	5

Food exchanges per ¾-cup serving: 1 BREAD, ½ MILK, ½ lean MEAT, 1 FAT

Squash with Apples

1   pound winter squash (acorn, butternut, or
    Hubbard), peeled and seeded
1   large baking apple, peeled
¼   cup water
1   tablespoon diet margarine
1   tablespoon fresh lemon juice
1   tablespoon molasses
4   packets artificial sweetener (Equal)
¼   teaspoon ground cinnamon
⅛   teaspoon ground nutmeg

1. Cut squash and apple into ½-inch cubes.
2. Put squash and apple into large skillet with water,
   margarine, and lemon juice over medium-high heat.
   Cover and cook, stirring occasionally, until just tender
   and liquid is absorbed.
3. Stir in molasses, sweetener, and spices.

Yield: 4 ½-cup servings

Nutritive values per ½-cup serving:	CAL	CHO (gm)	PRO (gm)	FAT (gm)
	109	24	1	1

Food exchanges per ½-cup
serving: 1 BREAD, 1 FRUIT, trace FAT

Oven-Fried Squash

½ cup cornmeal
½ teaspoon salt
¼ teaspoon freshly ground pepper
1 egg
3 tablespoons nonfat yogurt
3 medium yellow squash or zucchini, cut
  into ¼-inch slices
  Lemon wedges

1. Preheat oven to 350°F.
2. Combine cornmeal, salt, and pepper; set aside. Combine egg and yogurt; beat well. Dip squash in egg mixture; dredge in cornmeal.
3. Place squash in a nonstick baking pan in a single layer. Bake for 30–40 minutes, until golden, turning once. Serve with lemon wedges.

Yield: 6 ⅓-cup servings

Nutritive values per ⅓-cup serving:	CAL	CHO (gm)	PRO (gm)	FAT (gm)
	69	12	3	1

Food exchanges per ⅓-cup
serving: ½ BREAD, 1 VEGETABLE, trace
FAT

NONSTARCHY VEGETABLES

Cauliflower or Broccoli Parmesan

Here's an easy way to add some zest to these vegetables.

> 1 pound broccoli or cauliflower
> 2 tablespoons water for microwave *or* ¼ cup water for steaming
> 1 tablespoon diet margarine, melted
> Juice of ½ lemon
> 2 tablespoons minced fresh parsley
> Freshly ground white pepper
> 2 tablespoons grated Parmesan cheese

1. Cut tough stem ends off broccoli. Cut into long-stemmed flowerets (they look like trees to some children). Do the same for cauliflower (only shorter!).
2. For microwaving, put vegetables into 1-quart casserole with 2 tablespoons water and cover with plastic. Cook on HIGH for 5 minutes. Let stand for 3–4 minutes. Test with fork to see if it's tender. Broccoli should still be bright green. For steaming, place ¼ cup water in saucepan. Bring to boil. Use a steamer basket if you have one. Cover and steam for 5 minutes. Let stand, covered, for 3–4 minutes.
3. Drizzle margarine over vegetables in a serving dish. Squeeze lemon over and top with parsley, pepper, and cheese. Serve.

Yield: 4 ¾-cup servings

Nutritive values per ¾-cup serving:	CAL	CHO (gm)	PRO (gm)	FAT (gm)
	54	6	3	2

Food exchanges per ¾-cup serving: 1 VEGETABLE, ½ FAT

Sesame Broccoli

I prepare broccoli at least once a week. It's one of the most nutritious vegetables you can eat. Broccoli is a member of the cabbage family. Cabbage family members also include cauliflower, Brussels sprouts, kale, turnip greens, and kohlrabi. They contain sub-stances called indoles *that help protect cells from damage by cancer-causing chemicals. Broccoli is also an excellent source of vitamin C, vitamin A, and fiber.*

1   1½-pound bunch broccoli
½   teaspoon sesame oil
1   tablespoon sesame seeds
1   teaspoon peanut oil
1   clove garlic, minced
6   green onions, chopped
½   cup sliced water chestnuts (optional)
1   tablespoon dry sherry
1   tablespoon soy sauce
2   tablespoons water

1. Trim leaves off broccoli. Remove tough ends of lower stalks. Cut into flowerets and cut peeled stem into ¼-inch slices.
2. Heat sesame oil in wok or large skillet until hot. Toast sesame seeds until they start to turn golden. Remove and set aside.
3. Add peanut oil to wok with garlic and onions. Stir-fry for 1 minute.
4. Add broccoli slices and stir-fry for 3 minutes. Add flowerets and remaining ingredients. Reduce heat, cover, and steam for 5 minutes. Sprinkle sesame seeds over and serve.

Variation
Add 3 medium carrots, sliced, with broccoli slices and ¼ head green cabbage, chopped, with flowerets.

Yield: 6 ¾-cup servings

Nutritive values per ¾-cup serving:	CAL	CHO (gm)	PRO (gm)	FAT (gm)
	71	8	3	3

Food exchanges per ¾-cup
serving: 1½ VEGETABLE, ½ FAT

Nutritive values Variation per ¾-cup serving:	CAL	CHO (gm)	PRO (gm)	FAT (gm)
	96	13	5	3

Food exchanges Variation per
¾-cup serving: 2½ VEGETABLE, ½ FAT

Tart Red Cabbage

This can be served hot or cold.

½ cup red wine
½ cup red wine vinegar
½ teaspoon ground cinnamon
1 small onion, chopped
1 small head red cabbage (about 1–1½
    pounds), shredded
2 medium apples, sliced thin

Combine wine, vinegar, and cinnamon in large, heavy
saucepan. Heat to boil and reduce heat. Add onion, cabbage, and apples. Simmer for 1½ hours, covered. Add a
little water if necessary.

Yield: 6 ½-cup servings

Nutritive values per ½-cup serving:	CAL	CHO (gm)	PRO (gm)	FAT (gm)
	68	15	2	0

Food exchanges per ½-cup
serving: 1 FRUIT, 1 VEGETABLE

Sautéed Cabbage

Cabbage is rich in fiber, potassium, and vitamin C. Add shredded red or green cabbage to salads for extra nutrition.

1   1½-pound head green cabbage
1   shallot, minced, *or* ¼ small onion, minced
1   tablespoon minced fresh parsley
    Freshly ground pepper to taste
½   cup homemade chicken stock
½   teaspoon fennel seeds

1. With a sharp knife, cut out most of the core of the cabbage, leaving just enough to hold the head together. Slice the head into wedges about 1½ inches thick.

2. Put the cabbage, shallot, parsley, pepper, and stock in a large skillet. Cover and cook the cabbage over moderate heat for about 12 minutes, basting it several times with the pan juices.

3. When the cabbage is nearly done, sprinkle it with fennel seeds. Serve the cabbage with a little of the pan juices.

Yield: 6 ½-cup servings

Nutritive values per ½-cup serving:	CAL	CHO (gm)	PRO (gm)	FAT (gm)
	28	5	2	0

Food exchanges per ½-cup serving: 1 VEGETABLE

Fruit Spiced Carrots

1   pound carrots, without tops
¼ cup water
½ cup unsweetened orange or pineapple juice
½ teaspoon ground cinnamon
¼ teaspoon ground nutmeg
1   teaspoon grated orange or lemon zest

1. Cut carrots into ¼-inch slices. Combine water and juice with carrots in a medium saucepan. Bring to a boil. Cover and simmer for 20 minutes, until tender.

2. Stir in spices and zest.

Variation
Cook carrots in water and drain. Sprinkle with 1 table-spoon diet margarine, melted, juice of ½ lemon, and 1 packet Equal. Stir and serve.

Yield: 8 ½-cup servings

Nutritive values per ½-cup serving:	CAL	CHO (gm)	PRO (gm)	FAT (gm)
	28	5	2	0

Food exchanges per ½-cup serving:	1 VEGETABLE			

Cucumber Salad

4 cucumbers, peeled and sliced
4 green onions, chopped
¼ cup chopped fresh parsley
1 teaspoon dried dillweed
½ teaspoon basil leaves
1 clove garlic, minced or pressed
1 tablespoon dark sesame oil
½ cup rice vinegar

Put all ingredients into a bowl. Mix lightly and refrigerate 2–3 hours before serving.

Yield: 8 ½-cup servings

Nutritive values per ½-cup serving:	CAL	CHO (gm)	PRO (gm)	FAT (gm)
	21	3	0	1

Food exchanges per ½-cup serving: ½ VEGETABLE, trace FAT

Continental Green Beans

I love green beans raw, and my boys will sometimes eat them with dip. You can steam them for 5 minutes (they should still be bright green) or try this easy recipe.

1 16-ounce bag frozen green beans, defrosted, *or* 1 pound fresh, trimmed
1 6-ounce can tomato juice
½ small onion, minced
1 teaspoon oregano leaves
¼ teaspoon freshly ground pepper
1 tablespoon grated Parmesan cheese

Combine all ingredients except cheese in a saucepan. Simmer, covered, for 3 minutes. Uncover and simmer until liquid is almost gone. Sprinkle with cheese.

Yield: 4 ½-cup servings

Nutritive values per ½-cup serving:	CAL	CHO (gm)	PRO (gm)	FAT (gm)
	48	9	3	0

Food exchanges per ½-cup serving: 2 VEGETABLE

Baked Spinach

This recipe is an adaptation of one I found in The Art of Cooking for the Diabetic, *by Katharine Middleton and Mary Abbott Hess (Contemporary Books, 1978).*

2 eggs, beaten
1 tablespoon flour
¼ teaspoon salt
⅛ teaspoon freshly ground pepper
1 small clove garlic, minced
½ teaspoon ground nutmeg
1 tablespoon fresh lemon juice
2 10-ounce packages frozen chopped spinach, defrosted
½ teaspoon olive oil

1. Preheat oven to 350°F.
2. Beat eggs and add flour, salt, pepper, garlic, nutmeg, and lemon juice. Beat well. Add spinach and mix.
3. Oil 1-quart casserole with olive oil. Pour mixture in and bake for 20–25 minutes.

Yield: 5 ½-cup servings

Nutritive values per ½-cup serving:	CAL	CHO (gm)	PRO (gm)	FAT (gm)
	54	5	4	2

Food exchanges per ½-cup serving: 1 VEGETABLE, ½ FAT

Stir-Fry Squash

1 pound yellow squash or zucchini
2 teaspoons peanut oil
2 green onions, sliced
1 teaspoon soy sauce
1 teaspoon sugar
2 tablespoons water

1. Cut squash in half lengthwise, then diagonally into ¼-inch slices.
2. Heat peanut oil in a wok or heavy skillet over high heat. Add onions and stir-fry for a few seconds. Add squash and cook, stirring, for 1 minute.
3. Add soy sauce, sugar, and water. Stir well. Cover and cook over medium heat for 3 minutes. Serve.

Yield: 4 ⅔-cup servings

Nutritive values per ⅔-cup serving:	CAL	CHO (gm)	PRO (gm)	FAT (gm)
	50	6	2	2

Food exchanges per ⅔-cup
serving: 1 VEGETABLE, ½ FAT

Zucchini Italiano

3 cups sliced zucchini (approximately 1
   pound)
1 cup homemade chicken broth
1 6-ounce can tomato paste
1 onion, chopped
1 teaspoon oregano leaves
1 teaspoon basil leaves
1 clove garlic, minced
1 tablespoon bread crumbs
2 tablespoons grated Parmesan cheese

1. Preheat oven to 350°F.
2. Combine zucchini, broth, tomato paste, onion, herbs,
and garlic in casserole. Sprinkle with crumbs and
cheese. Bake, uncovered, for 1 hour or until tender.

Yield: 6 ½-cup servings

Nutritive values per ½-cup serving:	CAL	CHO (gm)	PRO (gm)	FAT (gm)
	48	9	3	0

Food exchanges per ½-cup
serving: 2 VEGETABLE

Swiss Chard Sauté

This is a tasty way to prepare this healthy green. If your child won't eat it, eat it yourself and make a fuss about how good it is! Both Swiss chard and kale are rich in calcium and vitamins A and C.

    1 teaspoon sesame oil or olive oil
    1 teaspoon minced garlic
    ½ cup thinly sliced onion
    ⅔ cup sliced celery
    1 tablespoon water
    4 cups coarsely chopped Swiss chard or kale
       Freshly ground black pepper
    1 tablespoon red wine vinegar

1. Heat the oil in a large skillet (preferably nonstick) and add the garlic, onion, and celery. Sauté, stirring, for about 3 minutes

2. Add the water and the Swiss chard. Season the mixture with pepper, stirring the ingredients to combine them well. Cover the pan and simmer the mixture, stirring it occasionally, over low heat for about 5 minutes or until the chard is wilted and tender. Sprinkle vinegar over the mixture.

Yield: 4 ½-cup servings

Nutritive values per ½-cup serving:	CAL	CHO (gm)	PRO (gm)	FAT (gm)
	62	8	3	2

Food exchanges per ½-cup
serving: 1½ VEGETABLE, ½ FAT

Mashed Turnips

These two recipes are good ways to prepare turnips that children will enjoy because they masquerade as potatoes!

> 1 pound turnips, peeled and diced
> 2 cups boiling water
> 1 tablespoon diet margarine
> ½ teaspoon salt
> ¼ teaspoon freshly ground pepper
> ¼ teaspoon ground nutmeg
> Paprika

1. Add turnips to boiling water in a saucepan. Lower heat, cover, and cook 20 minutes, until tender. Drain.
2. Mash turnips, adding margarine and seasonings. Sprinkle some paprika on top.

Yield: 4 ½-cup servings

Nutritive values per ½-cup serving:	CAL	CHO (gm)	PRO (gm)	FAT (gm)
	41	7	1	1

Food exchanges per ½-cup serving:	1½ VEGETABLE

Hash Brown Turnips

1   pound turnips, peeled and diced
1   teaspoon olive oil
½   cup chopped onion
¼   teaspoon salt
¼   teaspoon freshly ground pepper
¼   teaspoon powdered sage
¼   teaspoon thyme leaves

1. Cook turnips in a covered saucepan in boiling water to cover, about 20 minutes, until tender. Drain.
2. Heat oil in skillet over medium-high heat. Add all ingredients and cook, stirring occasionally, until turnips are lightly browned.

Yield: 4 ½-cup servings

Nutritive values per ½-cup serving:	CAL	CHO (gm)	PRO (gm)	FAT (gm)
	49	8	2	1

Food exchanges per ½-cup serving: 1½ VEGETABLE

Chinese Vegetables

I serve this with the Oriental Flank Steak earlier in this chapter (see index for recipe). It's one of my boys' favorite dinners. Bok choy looks like a cross between celery and spinach and is available in many large supermarkets. It is a good source of calcium and vitamin A. It is a member of the cabbage family and contains cancer-blocking agents.

1   teaspoon dark sesame oil
1   clove garlic, minced
1   teaspoon seeded and minced fresh
    gingerroot
2   stalks celery, chopped
4   green onions, chopped
1   green pepper, cut into strips
6   water chestnuts, sliced
½   pound fresh Chinese pea pods, stemmed
1   bunch bok choy, cut across the stalk in
    shreds
2   teaspoons soy sauce
2   tablespoons cream sherry
2   tablespoons chicken stock or water

1. Heat oil in wok or large skillet and stir-fry garlic and ginger over medium-high heat for 1 minute.
2. Add remaining ingredients, turn heat to high, and stir-fry for 3–4 minutes. Turn heat off, cover, and let steam for 2 minutes. Serve.

Variation
Use ½ head green cabbage, shredded, instead of bok choy, and 2 small zucchini instead of celery, cut into julienne strips. Add 1 medium tomato, chopped. (No real difference in exchanges.)

Yield: 6 ¾-cup servings

Nutritive values per serving:	CAL	CHO (gm)	PRO (gm)	FAT (gm)
	44	8	3	0
Food exchanges per serving:	1½ VEGETABLE			

Skillet Vegetables

This recipe is great served many different ways. Serve it over brown rice for a complete meal, or add extra chili powder and serve it on a flour tortilla, or serve it as is, for a tasty vegetable side dish.

1 large onion, chopped
1 clove garlic, minced
3 small zucchini, sliced
3 carrots, sliced thin
2 stalks celery, sliced thin
1 cup broccoli flowerets
1 cup cauliflower pieces
1 cup frozen corn kernels
1 16-ounce can tomatoes
1 teaspoon basil leaves
1 teaspoon chili powder
1 cup shredded sharp cheddar cheese

1. Place all vegetables in large, heavy skillet, breaking up tomatoes into small pieces.
2. Add seasonings. Cover and simmer for 45 minutes to 1 hour, until tender. Put cheese on top, cover, and cook until cheese melts, 2–3 minutes.

Yield: 8 ⅔-cup servings

Nutritive values per ⅔-cup serving:	CAL	CHO (gm)	PRO (gm)	FAT (gm)
	117	11	7	5

Food exchanges per ⅔-cup serving: ½ high-fat MEAT, 2 VEGETABLE

Tangy Buttermilk Dressing

This is similar to ranch-style dressing, but it's a free food!

³⁄₄ cup buttermilk (from skim milk)
1 tablespoon prepared horseradish (no added sugar)
1 tablespoon fresh lemon juice
1 packet artificial sweetener (Equal)
1 tablespoon Dijon mustard
1 teaspoon dried dillweed
2 tablespoons minced fresh parsley

Blend all ingredients together.

Yield: 1 cup

Nutritive values per 2-tablespoon serving:	CAL	CHO (gm)	PRO (gm)	FAT (gm)
	8	1	1	0

Food exchanges per 2-tablespoon serving:	FREE up to ⅓ cup

Mock Thousand Island Dressing

¼ cup nonfat yogurt
¼ cup catsup or chili sauce
2 tablespoons wine vinegar or fresh lemon
juice
Freshly ground pepper to taste
⅛ teaspoon hot red pepper sauce
⅛ teaspoon garlic powder
½ teaspoon Worcestershire sauce

1. Combine all ingredients well.
2. Chill before serving on tossed greens.

Yield: ½ cup (4 servings)

Nutritive values per 2-tablespoon serving:	CAL	CHO (gm)	PRO (gm)	FAT (gm)
	24	6	0	0

Food exchanges per 2-tablespoon
serving: ½ BREAD

Creamy Vinaigrette

This is from Jane Brody's Good Food Book.

- ⅔ cup low-fat yogurt
- ⅓ cup apple cider vinegar
- 2 tablespoons olive oil
- 1 tablespoon Dijon mustard
- 1 tablespoon fresh lemon juice
- 1 very large clove garlic, crushed
- 1 tablespoon reduced-sodium soy sauce (optional)
- ¼ teaspoon dried dillweed

Combine all ingredients in a bowl or jar with a tight-fitting lid. Whisk or shake to blend well.

Yield: about 1¼ cups

Nutritive values per 2-tablespoon serving:	CAL	CHO (gm)	PRO (gm)	FAT (gm)
	35	1	1	3

Food exchanges per 2-tablespoon serving: ½ FAT

Low-Calorie Mayonnaise

  1 cup low-fat cottage cheese or part-skim
     ricotta
  2 tablespoons fresh lemon juice
  2 egg yolks
  1 teaspoon Dijon mustard
  1 teaspoon dillweed or basil or chives
     (optional)
  ¼ teaspoon salt

Blend all ingredients in a blender or food processor until
they are smooth.

Yield: 1⅓ cup

Nutritive values per 1-tablespoon serving:	CAL	CHO (gm)	PRO (gm)	FAT (gm)
	61	0	4	5

Food exchanges per 1-tablespoon serving:	
	½ lean MEAT, ½ FAT

Gravy from Meat Drippings

Here's a low-calorie, low-fat gravy for your whole family.

> Skim milk, bouillon, water, or vegetable stock
> Meat drippings with fat removed*
> 2   tablespoons flour
> ¼   cup cold skim milk, bouillon, water, or vegetable stock
> Salt and pepper to taste

1. Add liquid to the drippings to make a total of ¾ cup.
2. Mix the flour with ¼ cup cold liquid.
3. Stir flour mixture into drippings mixture.
4. Heat, stirring constantly, until thickened.
5. Season to taste with salt and pepper.

Yield: 1 cup

Nutritive values per ¼-cup serving:	CAL	CHO (gm)	PRO (gm)	FAT (gm)
	16	4	0	0

Food exchanges per ¼-cup serving:	FREE

---

*To remove fat from drippings, pour drippings into a container. Chill in refrigerator (may be chilled quickly by putting in the freezer or adding an ice cube to the drippings). Remove solid fat that forms at the top. Store extra drippings in refrigerator or freezer for later use.

DESSERTS
Lemon Snow Pudding

Here's a free dessert! It's courtesy of The Art of Cooking for the Diabetic, *by Katharine Middleton and Mary Abbott Hess (Contemporary Books, 1978).*

> 1 tablespoon unflavored granulated gelatin
> ½ cup cold water
> 1 tablespoon grated lemon zest
> ¼ cup fresh lemon juice
> 1¼ cups boiling water
> 12 packets artificial sweetener (Equal)
> 2 medium egg whites
> ¼ teaspoon vanilla extract
> ¼ teaspoon lemon extract
> Grated lemon zest for garnish

1. Soak gelatin in cold water. Meanwhile, combine lemon zest, juice, and boiling water in a bowl. Add softened gelatin and sweetener; mix well. Chill until it is the consistency of unbeaten egg whites.
2. Add unbeaten egg whites, vanilla extract, and lemon extract. Beat with a rotary beater until it is very fluffy and holds its shape. Pile into 6 parfait glasses. Top with a little extra grated lemon zest.

Yield: 4 ½-cup servings

Nutritive values per serving:	This whole recipe is 32 calories and not quite 1 lean MEAT
Food exchanges per serving:	FREE up to 2 cups

Chocolate Delight

1 envelope unflavored gelatin
2 tablespoons unsweetened cocoa powder
2 eggs, separated
2 cups skim milk
1½ teaspoons vanilla extract
12 packets artificial sweetener (Equal)

1. In a medium saucepan, mix unflavored gelatin with cocoa. Beat egg yolks with 1 cup of the skim milk and add to saucepan. Let stand 1 minute.
2. Place saucepan over low heat and stir until gelatin is dissolved, about 5 minutes. Remove from heat. Add remaining cup of skim milk, plus vanilla and sweetener. Chill mixture in a large bowl, stirring occasionally, until slight mounds form when dropped from a spoon.
3. In a large bowl, beat egg whites at high speed until soft peaks form. Gradually add gelatin mixture and beat until mixture increases in volume, about 5 minutes.
4. Chill until slightly thickened. Turn into individual dishes or a 4-cup serving bowl. Chill until firm.

Yield: 8 ½-cup servings

Nutritive values per ½-cup serving:	CAL	CHO (gm)	PRO (gm)	FAT (gm)
	41	4	4	1

Food exchanges per ½-cup serving:	½ MILK, trace FAT

Chocolate Sauce

This recipe is from The New Diabetic Cookbook, *by Mabel Cavaiani (Contemporary Books, 1984). It's nice to have an alternative to fudge sauce that's appropriate for diabetics on special occasions.*

3 tablespoons unsweetened cocoa powder
1 tablespoon cornstarch
⅓ cup instant dry milk
⅛ teaspoon salt
1½ cups water
1 tablespoon margarine
2 teaspoons vanilla extract
12 packets artificial sweetener (Equal)

1. Stir together cocoa, cornstarch, dry milk, and salt to blend in a small saucepan. Stir water into dry mixture until smooth. Add margarine and cook and stir over low heat. Bring to a boil and simmer 2 minutes, stirring constantly. Remove from heat.
2. Add vanilla and sweetener to sauce. Stir lightly to mix. Pour into a glass jar and refrigerate until used. Return to room temperature before serving over ice cream or reheat to serve on cake or pudding.

Yield: 1½ cups (12 servings)

Nutritive values per 2-tablespoon serving:	CAL	CHO (gm)	PRO (gm)	FAT (gm)
	29	3	2	1

Food exchanges per 2-tablespoon serving: ¼ MILK, trace FAT

All-American Cranberry Sauce

The original recipe called for 1½ cups of maple syrup. I played around with it and came up with the following. After you taste it, I doubt you will ever use canned cranberry sauce again!

1 12-ounce bag fresh cranberries, sorted and washed
¼ cup real maple syrup
1 cup water
2 teaspoons maple flavoring
1 tablespoon grated orange zest
¾ teaspoon ground ginger
2 teaspoons arrowroot
12 packets artificial sweetener (Equal)

1. In medium saucepan, combine cranberries, syrup, and water and bring to boil. Reduce heat and simmer for 5 minutes, until berries start to pop.
2. Add maple flavoring, orange zest, and ginger. Cook a few minutes. Stir in arrowroot and simmer until thickened. Stir in sweetener. Mix thoroughly. Cool and refrigerate.

Yield: 2 cups (16 servings)

Nutritive values per 2-tablespoon serving:	CAL	CHO (gm)	PRO (gm)	FAT (gm)
	24	6	0	0

Food exchanges per 2-tablespoon serving: ½ FRUIT

Cranberry Relish

1 12-ounce package fresh cranberries, washed and drained
1 orange, seeded
1 apple, cored
8 packets artificial sweetener (Equal)

Place a small amount of cranberries, a slice of orange, and a slice of apple in a blender or food processor and chop coarsely. Repeat until all ingredients are chopped. Add sweetener. Mix well and chill overnight.

Yield: 12 ¼-cup servings

Nutritive values per ¼-cup serving:	CAL	CHO (gm)	PRO (gm)	FAT (gm)
	24	6	0	0

Food exchanges per ¼-cup serving:

½ FRUIT (up to 4 tablespoons FREE)

Cranberry Mold

This is another adaptation of what is normally a highly caloric recipe.

   1   12-ounce bag fresh cranberries
   1   orange
   1   3-ounce package sugar-free lemon gelatin
   1   3-ounce package sugar-free raspberry gelatin
   2   cups boiling water
   1   20-ounce can unsweetened crushed pineapple in juice
   ½   cup chopped walnuts
   1   teaspoon peeled and grated fresh gingerroot *or* ½ teaspoon ground ginger
   12 packets artificial sweetener (Equal)

1. Grind cranberries in food processor until fine. Cut thin strips of peel off the orange. Chop orange pulp and add peel and pulp to processor and chop again. Set aside.
2. Combine gelatins with boiling water. Add remaining ingredients and cranberry mixture. Mix well. Chill until set in large mold or 9- by 13-inch pan.

Yield: 12 ¾-cup servings

Nutritive values per ¾-cup serving:	CAL	CHO (gm)	PRO (gm)	FAT (gm)
	71	10	1	3

Food exchanges per ¾-cup serving:	1 FRUIT, ½ FAT

Cran-Apple Crisp

2 medium tart apples, sliced (about 3 cups)
1½ cups fresh cranberries
¼ cup unsweetened orange juice
1 tablespoon grated orange zest
⅓ cup unbleached white flour
⅓ cup quick oats, uncooked
¼ cup Brown SugarTwin
1 teaspoon ground cinnamon
¼ teaspoon ground nutmeg
2 tablespoons corn or safflower oil

1. Preheat oven to 375°F.
2. In medium bowl, combine apples, cranberries, orange juice, and zest. Place in shallow 1½-quart baking dish.
3. In medium bowl, combine flour, oats, Brown Sugar-Twin, cinnamon, nutmeg, and oil until crumbly. Sprinkle over apple mixture. Bake 25 minutes or until apples are tender and topping is golden. Serve warm.

Yield: 6 ¾-cup servings

Nutritive values per ¾-cup serving:	CAL	CHO (gm)	PRO (gm)	FAT (gm)
	128	22	1	4

Food exchanges per ¾-cup
serving: ½ BREAD, 1½ FRUIT, 1 FAT

Easy Sugarless Pumpkin Pie

- 2 eggs, slightly beaten
- 1 16-ounce can pureed pumpkin
- 12 packets artificial sweetener (equal to ½ cup sugar)
- ½ teaspoon salt
- 1 teaspoon ground cinnamon
- ½ teaspoon ground ginger
- ¼ teaspoon ground cloves
- 1 teaspoon vanilla extract
- 1 12-ounce can evaporated skim milk
- 1 9-inch unbaked homemade pie crust (Lean Pie Crust; see index) or frozen pie shell

1. Preheat oven to 425°F.
2. Combine filling ingredients in order given.
3. Pour into pie shell.
4. Bake 15 minutes. Reduce temperature to 350°F and bake an additional 45 minutes or until knife inserted near center of pie comes out clean.

Yield: 1 9-inch pie (8 servings)

Nutritive values per serving:	CAL	CHO (gm)	PRO (gm)	FAT (gm)
	176	29	6	4

Food exchanges per serving: 1½ BREAD, ½ MILK, 1 FAT

PART III
THE COPEBOOK

None of us will ever forget the moment we were told that our child had diabetes. Our lives changed quickly. We were expected to learn all the complexities of living with diabetes, while handling our own sense of grief, guilt, and anger.

Many parents go through their first year after diagnosis feeling overwhelmed. One mother wrote me that eight months after her dauther's diagnosis she still found it difficult to get through a day without crying. She felt her depression over her daughter's diabetes would never end. In the meantime, her daughter was doing fine.

There's an element of this mother's sadness that is a significant factor not only in dealing with diabetes, but in dealing with life. That element is expectations.

We all have expectations. As we grow, we ought to be adjusting our expectations based on the realities we encounter. The expectation that our children will grow up to be healthy, happy, and unencumbered is a deep-seated dream of every parent. Diabetes alters our expectations. It demands not only that we make room in our lives for additional responsibilities and restrictions on a daily basis, but that we live with the possibility of our child's developing diabetic complications. It's a difficult adjustment to make.

That's why I've written this section. As a parent, I know how vital it is to have input from other parents of children with diabetes, to know you're not alone. "Perspective" will help you understand what to expect, physically and psychologically, from your child. "Specifics" answers many common questions parents have. "Resources" will help you know where to look for help. Finally, "Research" will give you what we, as parents, need most—hope for the future.

"The Copebook" is based on interviews with parents and experts. It has been written under the guidance of Dr. Jonathan Kellerman. Dr. Kellerman is a clinical associate professor of pediatrics at the USC School of Medicine. He's also the cofounder and former director of the Psychosocial Program at Children's Hospital in Los Angeles. He has been involved for years in government and private studies of children with chronic illness.

Researching and writing this section has expanded my understanding of my own children and deepened my personal resources. It has helped me become a more sensitive parent. I know it will help you.

10
Perspective

As parents of diabetic children, we have a lot that concerns us. We worry about our child's food, insulin, and exercise. We also worry about how the stress of dealing with a chronic illness will affect our child socially and psychologically. Will it change or ruin her life? Yes and no. It will alter many elements of your child's life, but there is no reason your child can't grow up to be as emotionally and psychologically healthy as anyone else.

This was not always thought to be the case. There used to be the opinion among health professionals that chronically ill children would automatically have psychological problems. Well, that's not true. In one study conducted by Dr. Kellerman and his associates, adolescents with diabetes, cancer, and cystic fibrosis were compared with a matched group of teenagers without any illnesses. The tests were based on standardized psychological measures. Both groups were found to be basically the same. In each group, most of them were well adjusted and some had problems. So, the fact that your child is chronically ill doesn't mean she will have emotional problems. She can grow up to be as stable and fulfilled as anyone else.

However, diabetes doesn't make it easy! It is actually one of the most difficult diseases because of all the demands it makes on a child's behavior. Many illnesses are passive ones. You receive treatment; you take your medication. Your doctor makes the decisions and you merely follow directions. Diabetes, on the other hand, lays it all in your lap. It necessitates learning to be your own doctor. It demands constant awareness and discipline.

302 KIDS, FOOD, AND DIABETES

One of the major psychological issues of childhood is learning control and mastery of one's life. For that matter, the whole process of human development is one of gaining control. (Heaven knows, I'm still working on it!) Look how difficult it is for most adults to stay on a strict diet or stop smoking. Yet, we expect an eight- or nine-year-old to stick to his diet every hour of every day. Clearly, that means asking a child to engage in a level of self-control for which he is not equipped.

I remember what one doctor recommended to parents who are being unrealistic. He suggested they follow their child's diet plan plus give themselves blood tests and injections of sterile water whenever their child did. Most of the parents couldn't stay on it for more than a few days. It helped them understand what their children go through.

Another path to understanding is by knowing something about child development and by sharpening your communication skills. Communication involves listening, being sensitive to nonverbal signs, and having a willingness to understand, in addition to being willing and able to express your own feelings appropriately. In this chapter, you will find information and suggestions that may help you become more skillful in communicating with your child.

There is a certain rhythm to the way in which your child grows. There are periods of happiness and security that alternate with periods of disruption. Psychologists refer to these periods as *stages of equilibrium and disequilibrium*. These patterns are evident when we look at the characteristics of each age. Knowing these patterns can help you better understand the additional difficulty diabetes may present for you and your child.

The ages and descriptions are, of course, approximate and are not meant to be exact measurements. Each child is an individual and exemplifies these stages in his own way.

THE TODDLER:
AGE TWO TO FIVE

This is a very powerful stage of life. It's called the *first adolescence*. The toddler is just beginning to develop and express his sense of self. The king of egocentrics, he believes he is the origin of all actions in the universe. Cause and effect mean very little. Everything exists for the moment. He finds it difficult to consider more than one situation at a time. A child of this age can also have a strong sense of guilt. Since he believes he is the source of everything, illness and pain may be viewed as a punishment.

The two-year-old is at a stage of equilibrium. He runs and climbs surely. He uses language effectively to make his wants known and, because of that, suffers from much less frustration than as an infant. He likes to please others and is often loving and responsive. Age two-and-a-half changes all that. He becomes rigid and inflexible. He is demanding and wants to make all decisions himself. Since he has no ability to choose among alternatives, decisions are very difficult. It is an age of violent emotions.

At three, the resistance changes to conformity. The attitude becomes more easygoing and cooperative. People are important to him, and he is more willing to share. His increased ability with language makes him an interesting companion. He is pleased with himself and with those about him. At three-and-a-half, once again he enters a time of insecurity and disequilibrium. Lack of coordination is very characteristic of this age and may express itself as stumbling, falling, fear of heights, or stuttering. He's very emotionally insecure, too. He can be very demanding and extremely jealous. He needs extra patience and understanding.

Four is best described as "out of bounds." Everything he does is overboard. He hits, kicks, and throws things. He runs away. He's loud and silly or full of anger. He loves to use language to shock and loves to defy his parents. His imagination is boundless also, and he easily forgets the line between fantasy and reality. Four is a brash age. He needs to test himself and expand his world.

At four-and-a-half he begins to pull back a little. He becomes very concerned with what is real. He loves to discuss things in detail and likes to be shown. He is improving his control and perfecting his skills. He handles frustration a little better, too.

Five is a time of extreme balance, a good age. He's reliable, stable, and well adjusted. He likes to be instructed and to get permission. He means to do what's right and be a good boy. He's content and satisfied, and his parents are the center of his world.

These small children believe that their parents are all-powerful. Diabetic little ones sometimes think that their parents can take away their diabetes. It's important for your child to know that she didn't cause her diabetes and that, although you'd like to, you don't have the power to change it. A child at this age cannot make logical sense of detailed explanations about diabetes and its treatment, so you don't have to have all the answers. A matter-of-fact approach, a tone of confidence, and a spirit of "we'll handle this together" is most effective. Keep your explanation simple and as concrete as possible. Explain it in terms that your child can understand.

Brennan's father explained it this way: "You know Mommy and Daddy wear glasses to read and watch television. That's because our eyes don't work too well. You have something inside of you called a *pancreas* that also doesn't work too well. Instead of wearing glasses, you need to take shots of insulin so you'll feel good." Your attitude will strongly influence how your child feels about his diabetes.

I believe that diabetes is much harder on a parent than on the child at this stage. You alone know what diabetes is and can do. Your natural reaction may be one of gut-level fear. You may feel certain that if you're not at your child's side, watching over him every minute, something terrible will happen to him that no one else can properly handle. However, it is important to remember that the two- to five-year-old is at a tumultuous stage of striving for independence and autonomy. At the same time, he also has a deep fear of separation.

This is a time when your child needs loving reassurance, not excessive control and protectiveness. It's not easy to do when you're dealing with a disease as unpredictable as diabetes. It is further complicated if your child is so young that he can't recognize the feelings of an oncoming insulin reaction. Through careful observation you will come to know those signs and when reactions might possibly take place. One mother of a two-year-old noticed that her son's reactions were preceded by his feeling tired and his lying down—right on the spot—with his favorite bear. She laughingly told me, "The poor kid, every time he sat down or lay down, I gave him a blood test—bear or no bear!" It is important to help your child find a way to verbalize low blood sugar symptoms as early as possible. It might be "I feel funny" or "I'm low." Be sure to praise him for telling you.

Inherent in this quest for independence is a certain amount of necessary rebellion. Unfortunately for the parent of a diabetic, power struggles will often center around food. Try not to get into any battles. If your child won't eat one thing, try another. Finger foods, juice, or frozen yogurt bars or decorated foods may be appealing. There's nothing wrong with Cream of Wheat for dinner. Be flexible, but don't feel you've got to do a song and dance. Try not to pay extra attention if he's not eating.

Sometimes nothing you do will work. Rather than try to force-feed a fussy eater, you may just need to let the natural consequences occur. One of two things may happen: the lower blood sugar your child will experience may cause him to feel hungry (in which case your problem is solved), or your child may begin to have an insulin reaction. If you're watchful and prepared with glucose of some sort—juice, cake frosting in a tube—no harm will be done. After the reaction has subsided, you can talk to your child and explain why it happened and why it's important to eat at meal- and snacktimes. Sooner or later, your child needs to understand that not eating will cause him to feel bad. Don't scold or punish him. At any age, it may cause a child to lie or become evasive so as to avoid nagging. Work on positive reinforcement.

It's so hard to watch anything disturb or distress our children. It's normal to want to compensate for your child's diabetes, but try not to confuse security and affection with permissiveness and failure to set limits. Kids are smart (I'm sure you've noticed). One four-year-old has figured out how to stay up later. He can make his bedtime snack of a bowl of popcorn last for over an hour. When his mom says, "Finish up, or you'll go to bed without a snack," he says, "No, Mommy—I'm diabetic."

For the child who is too young to clearly communicate his feelings about diabetes, play therapy is a valuable tool that is used by professionals. Pounding wood, working with clay, and acting out with dolls or puppets can be creative outlets for your child's frustrations. When Brennan came home from the hospital after being diagnosed, he decided that his favorite doll, Joey, also had diabetes. He gave Joey shots for a while until the newness of it all wore off. I think it helped him feel a sense of control over diabetes by playing the role of the shot-giver, instead of just being the shot-receiver.

Also remember that these little ones can take things very literally. One child who had the flu had nightmares about bugs and monsters for weeks after the flu symptoms subsided. After much probing, it was discovered that this little boy had overheard his mother say that he "had a bug."

You need to keep checking to see how your child feels. You may have explained something once, but he may not have gotten it or remembered it. Role-playing can be very helpful to see how much your child understands and to assist in presenting further information. Be as concrete as possible. Use graphs or drawings if necessary. One six-year-old girl told her mother that when she came to Open House she'd easily be able to tell which drawing of the body was her daughter's. The mother was surprised to find that her daughter had hung an "out of order" sign where her pancreas would have been. That's one little girl with a sense of humor and a clear picture of what diabetes means.

Also, watch for signs of "acting out." A child who starts soiling his pants is giving you a message! Be aware that regressive behavior can often occur. If it's temporary, ignore it. If it continues, seek professional advice.

No matter how young your child is, seek ways to involve him in his diabetes care. Your little one can help choose the injection site, wipe the skin with alcohol (or wash it with soap and water), or pinch up the skin. A small band-aid and a kiss can help make it "all better." Use positive reinforcement for blood tests and injections. A chart with little stickers or stars for cooperation can be very helpful. When you child accumulates a certain number of stickers, you could plan some special activity.

A few extra words about infants. The same basic advice that applies to toddlers also applies to infants. Extra watchfulness is necessary, of course, because infants have no ability to identify oncoming insulin reactions. Blood testing becomes all the more important because it gives you accurate information if you're unsure of your child's symptoms. You can use heels, toes, and earlobes if your baby's fingers become tender. Always have supplies for reactions nearby. Some parents keep them in almost every room of the house. Try to build a support system of family and friends to help you deal with your feelings. Being able to talk to another parent who has raised an infant with diabetes is very helpful.

Diabetes places many restrictions on your child. Aside from doing what is necessary to maintain acceptable blood sugar control, give your child the freedom to be like any other child. You may worry about insulin reactions or the future, but don't let your concerns put a damper on the joyful immediacy of your toddler's view. Allow permissible pleasures. Provide opportunities for your child to have some control. If she must eat her snack, don't ask her if she wants to eat. A "no" won't be acceptable, and you'll then have to take control by insisting she eat. Instead, give her a choice: "Do you want to eat _____ or _____ or _____?"

Providing choices helps build self-esteem and confidence, and that's a vital part of parenting, whether or not your child has diabetes.

THE MIDDLE YEARS: AGE SIX TO TEN

The six-year-old can be much like the two-and-a-half-year-old—an emotional extremist who wants to be the center of his world. He wants all of everything. It's a difficult time.

At seven he is more withdrawn, more likely to complain. A child of seven can be very demanding, especially with himself. He tends to feel people are against him, don't like him, are picking on him. He needs sympathy but not babying.

If seven withdraws from the world, eight meets it head on. He loves challenges and is filled with energy and enthusiasm. He can be dramatic, even self-disparaging if he feels he's failed. He expects much from himself and his relationships with others.

Nine lives more of his life within than the eight-year-old. He's more self-contained and self-sufficient. He also has a serious side. He tends to worry and can be overly anxious. He complains, and often these complaints take physical manifestations. He is very concerned about pain and discomfort.

Ten is one of the nicest ages. Ten is characterized by cheerful obedience. He's satisfied with parents, teachers,

and the world in general. He's straightforward and matter-of-fact.

The development of self-esteem is very important during these years. Your child needs to experience discipline,
responsibility, and independence. A child's self-concept
will also often develop in correlation to his body image.
Diabetes can certainly pose a threat to that self-image. It
can also be used to enhance self-esteem. Your focusing on
the positives, giving praise for a "job well done," helps
your child feel competent about his ability to handle his
diabetes.

Once again, the way you view your child will influence
his self-image. I remember how proud I had been of
Brennan's size and health as a baby. He was nine pounds
at birth and was hardly ever sick as a toddler. When he got
diabetes, I had to struggle with my image of him. At first,
I thought, "It's all changed. He's not perfect anymore." It
took me a while to see that he was still the child he was
before. The only thing that had changed was that his
pancreas didn't function normally. He was the same, yet
at the same time different.

The problem of feeling different is not easy for a child.
On the one hand, you want to reassure your child that she
is "not different," but adjusting to being diabetic includes
accepting the "differentness," being comfortable with her
uniqueness.

Family support is most important, but acceptance by
peers runs a very close second. The way your child's
diabetes is handled in the school setting will have a
powerful effect on your child's feelings about herself.

There are some people who must know about your
child's diabetes and some who don't have to. All of your
child's caretakers need to be educated—the teachers,
school nurse, cafeteria manager, and bus driver, to name
a few. They need to know what happens when your child
has an insulin reaction. You should make sure they have
juice, crackers, and glucose tablets or cake-gel available at
all times to treat a reaction. You might want to keep some

blood-testing equipment with the school nurse. Talk with each of these people face to face.

Both JDF and ADA have pamphlets available that explain diabetes to teachers and other school personnel. Sometimes you can encounter resistance to your child's keeping blood-testing equipment at school. One mother was told they were worried it had something to do with drugs and drug abuse. Some people fear diabetes because they don't understand it. If necessary, get your doctor to send a letter to the school stating that the blood-testing equipment is an essential element of your child's care.

One mother arranged a small group meeting and showed a video presentation called *Teacher's Responsibility* (see index). She felt it had a very positive effect on the understanding and support her child received. Another mom signed up as room-mother so she could help influence the foods for class parties and snacktime. At one school, where no morning snack was served, one parent sent in graham crackers for all the kids so that her daughter wouldn't be singled out as the only one having a snack. You can decide with your child and her teacher how to handle snacks inconspicuously.

It's your child's decision to tell her classmates she has diabetes. Some children have no problem with it. One little girl, Brooke, brought her blood-testing equipment in for Show-and-Tell. Another boy presented a science report about diabetes to his class that caused a classmate to raise his hand and say, "I had diarrhea once, too." Some kids use the buddy system and have one classmate who knows about diabetes and watches out for reactions.

Most kids will be understanding and very impressed with your child's bravery once they know that diabetes means daily shots and blood tests. Some, however, can be obnoxious. Teach your child to be assertive. She might say something like, "My body has trouble with the way it handles sugar. I have to watch what I eat, test my blood several times, and give myself two shots every day. Could you do that?" If the teasing continues, she should ignore it or possibly enlist the aid of a teacher. There's a book that does a good job of explaining it in language a child can understand. It's called *You Can't Catch Diabetes from a Friend*, by Lynne Kipnis and Susan Adler (Triad Scientific Publishers, 1979).

Your child can participate in blood tests and shots from toddlerhood on up. Around the age of eight or nine, many diabetic kids will occasionally begin giving their own shots. They should be encouraged and closely supervised. These acts of gaining a sense of control over diabetes will add to your child's self esteem.

Don't be unrealistic in your expectations. The world of this child is still now-oriented. He can be logical and understand what diabetes is but does not really have the capacity to anticipate long-term complications. Your child is not going to stick to his diet all the time. Peer pressure and feelings of denial are common causes of "cheating." Remember that these dietary indiscretions are reinforced in part by the absence of any immediate ill effects. Having a higher than normal blood sugar doesn't feel bad. Rejection, nagging, and threats of complications are mostly ineffective and can often cause kids to lie to their parents. Try to emphasize the "can haves," not the "can't haves." Concentrate on permissible foods and work an occasional dessert into the insulin dosage. Also, teach your child how to figure treats into his diet.

At this age, support groups and summer camps are additional opportunities for your child to experience a sense of control and togetherness with other kids with diabetes. I heard about one group of diabetics at summer camp who decided that they didn't want to do individual urine tests any longer. They told their counselor they'd all pee into a barrel and that he could average it out! Brennan recently made friends with another boy, Adam, who has diabetes. I took them out to dinner, and, since Brennan was sitting across the table from me, Adam said he'd help Brennan give himself his shot. When they'd finished, Brennan said, "It's nice to have a friend with diabetes." What an understatement!

ADOLESCENCE: AGE 11 TO 16

Eleven is assertive, curious, and sociable. He's on the go. He may seem to be hungry all the time. He talks and talks. He is intense and is subject to variable moods. His whole being is in a process of growth and reorganization.

Twelve is less insistent, more reasonable, more companionable. She is in a stage of widening awareness. Less self-centered, she is outgoing and cooperative. Twelve is trying to grow up. Her peer group plays an important role in shaping her attitudes and interests. She exhibits an increased self-insight and self-control along with a greater sense of perspective.

Thirteen withdraws to some extent. Not always communicative, he may have spells of silence. He worries a great deal. It is a time of taking in, mulling over. He is not retreating from reality. He is probing, questioning, reflecting. He is more discriminating about the friends he chooses and the way he looks.

Fourteen is robust and expressive. She has a new self-assurance and is better oriented to both herself and her environment. She enjoys life. She also enjoys a better relationship with her parents. There is more mutual respect and understanding. She is anxious to be popular and sensitive about deviations from the norm.

Fifteen becomes more thoughtful. He may even seem indifferent. He is frugal with his energy and may be considered lazy or at least tired. He makes an effort to find just the right words to express himself and is concerned with precision. His moods are not as intense as they were at 13. His development at this age is marked by increasing self-awareness, independence, and loyalty to home, school, and community.

Sixteen is self-assured. She has achieved a sense of independence. She has many friends and usually prefers their company to the company of the family. She is more aware of the future than ever before and has strong feelings about marriage and career. Sixteen is generally well balanced. She is not touchy and covers hurt feelings.

She is more willing to see another person's view. She is, at this age, a prototype of a preadult.

It's very difficult to be a teenager and a diabetic. Diabetes does not fit in at all with what teenagers want. One teenaged boy who refused to keep his diabetes in control said succinctly, "Diabetes doesn't fit into my lifestyle."

Adolescents are obsessed with controlling their own life, defining their identity. This involves a great deal of experimentation and rebellion. It is a difficult time for most parents as it is, but add diabetes and the difficult becomes seemingly impossible.

Even though teenagers have the maturity to understand long-term ramifications of present actions, they really don't take it seriously or at least don't want to think about it all the time. Keeping the lines of communication open is very important. Nagging and threats just don't work and can actually be counterproductive.

The teen years are marked by spontaneity. Diabetes asks a teenager to limit much of that spontaneity by calculating and planning even the most basic activities such as eating and drinking. (I discuss handling alcohol and your child in Chapter 11.) Deciding to have pizza at the last minute after a football game is a normal activity for teens but for your child can mean a very high blood sugar. The key to control is knowledge and flexibility. That flexibility might be provided, for example, by being on three shots instead of two. That way, your teen could figure the pizza into a nighttime insulin dose. He could decide how much pizza he wants to eat and work out a formula ahead of time with his doctor or dietitian. Each piece of pizza is approximately two BREAD, and he might know that for two pieces (four BREAD) he might need to take two extra units of regular insulin. He can go off to the bathroom, if he wishes to keep it secret, take his shot, and then eat like everyone else. You and your teen can work out a way with the doctor to make diabetes fit your teenager's life. Self-discipline and responsibility will give him the control and freedom he desires.

On the other hand, a badly controlled diabetic teen may spend time having reactions, which can be embarrassing in front of friends. Hopefully, those episodes may provide a vivid example of the psychological value of good control.

In spite of this, your teenager may test the limits of not paying attention to his diabetes. It will frighten you. Testing limits is what being a teenager is all about. He defines what he is and is not by testing and rebelling against almost everything in his world. For some teens, these years are more difficult than for others. But whatever the degree of compliance, there is really not much you can do about it directly. You cannot stand over your teen's shoulder every minute and monitor everything he does. You cannot stop your teen from doing something self-destructive. It's part of the essential powerlessness of being a parent. Knowing that doesn't make it any easier, but at least you should be realistic. For a moment put yourself in your teen's shoes. He has an illness that is permanent, may maim or kill him, and requires daily, hourly concern and care. He faces the constant struggle between satisfying his immediate desires and knowing his long-term health may be at stake. That's a struggle for anyone, much less someone going through the disruptive forces of the teenage years.

It's his disease, and the sooner you encourage your child to "own" his diabetes, the better. That doesn't mean you wash your hands of it, because we parents know that's impossible. There is much you can do to guide and support positive behavior. Give him as much knowledge as possible. Consider yourself a consultant. Discuss the choices together and let your teen decide what to do whenever possible. See if your adolescent can describe how he sees your role in his diabetes care. How does he want you to help? Let him know how you view your role and negotiate the differences. Get professional help if you have trouble resolving them.

Concerning school, make sure your teen's teachers know about his diabetes. One teen I know of didn't bother to tell one of his teachers. When he "fell asleep" at his desk, his teacher decided to see how long he would sleep. Finally, when he could not be awakened, the paramedics were called, and his reaction was treated.

Also get your child and yourself involved in support groups and diabetes organizations. Karen Hostetler has headed up the Juvenile Diabetes Foundation chapter in Cleveland and founded a POLO (Parents of Little Ones) group there. She has noticed that over the years the parents who brought their children with them to the meetings seem to have fewer problems with compliance when adolescence hits. The parents who left their kids at home (they were "doing fine") are now calling because they don't know what to do with their diabetic teenagers.

This is possibly explained by these kids' knowing that they're not alone. They meet other diabetics at these meetings, hear others talk about how hard it is, and have a place where someone really understands. They also learn how to gain control of their diabetes. Control makes them feel good about themselves. The more knowledge about diabetes one has, the better. Blood glucose monitoring gives immediate feedback for better control. The feeling of being master of one's body and destiny is a powerful motivator. Give your child all the knowledge you can. Thanks to research, there is much good news about diabetes these days. Discussions about career, marriage, having children, and drinking alcohol can give valuable information and help allay fears.

If all else fails, ask for help. You deserve all the assistance you can get. Don't be afraid or embarrassed to ask a professional therapist to assist you in dealing with these difficult years. Almost every parent of a teen, with or without diabetes, feels there are times when he or she could use a little professional help. You won't necessarily get your child to do everything your way, but that's not the aim of counseling. Its purpose is to get the lines of communication open. Studies and professional observation have shown that families with good communication skills are more likely to get compliance from their diabetic teens. The love and trust that are important to any child are just as vital to your diabetic child.

ADVICE FROM PARENTS

Raising a child is a complicated procedure. A chronic illness like diabetes makes it even more difficult. It's frightening. You're not sure if you're doing a good job, if you're up to the challenge. As a parent, you need and deserve all the help you can get. Don't be afraid to ask for assistance if you need it. Enlist your family, friends, and neighbors. As one mother said, "It's nothing to be ashamed of. Most people are willing to help, in some way, if you just ask."

Remember, your child is a child first and a diabetic child second. Give your child all the tools and knowledge to regulate her diabetes so that she is the one in control. Give her the freedom to make mistakes while giving her as much responsibility as she is capable of handling.

Having diabetes means walking a fine line between controlling it and letting it control you. It's more than just physical control. Feelings are important. Expressing and sharing what hurts us somehow lessens its effect. Listen to your child's feelings. You don't have to have all the answers. You can't "fix" diabetes. Telling a child, "You could have something worse," doesn't help. She has diabetes, and that's bad enough as far as she is concerned. Talk about your feelings with your child. (Sometimes parents hide their feelings to protect their child. The child can pick up on this and may in turn hide her feelings.) Let her know she's loved. Remind her you're a team and you'll handle it together. Don't dwell on the "can't haves," or the "you should haves." Keep the lines of communication open. Studies have shown that there is a strong relationship between good parent-child relations and good control.

Good parent relations brings me to the subject of fathers and their involvement. It is very important that the father take an active role right from the beginning. If a dad is not knowledgeable or a part of a child's diabetes care, that child may think diabetes isn't very important.

Sibling cooperation is also a vital aspect of support. The education of all family members is essential. Siblings should be made to feel a part of the family effort to deal with diabetes. Helping treat an insulin reaction, assisting by distracting a younger diabetic child while a shot is given, or helping with blood tests reinforces family togetherness and helps discourage feelings of being left out. Diabetes is not easy for nondiabetic family members. I'll never forget the night of a JDF fundraiser in Bakersfield, California. I was conducting an auction from the stage and people were being very generous. Suddenly, I felt someone tug on my jacket and turned to see my then eight-year-old son, Robin. He handed me $5.00 and said, "I saved this from my allowance." Afterwards, I took him aside and praised him for his unselfish donation. With tears in his eyes, he said, "It was my only $5.00. I gave it to help diabetes research. You know, Brennan's diabetes is hard on me too."

"Oh, honey," I said. "Is it hard on you?"

"Yes, Brennan gets mad about having diabetes and beats me up."

I didn't know whether to laugh or cry.

I am a parent like you who knows what diabetes means. I know the hurt, the sense of loss. I know the frustration of wanting to take it all away, make it better, and not being able to do that. Talking with other parents helps. I want to share with you what some of the parents I interviewed asked me to tell you.

- "Trust yourself and your child. Knowing that you are the person who knows your child best is the real bottom line. No matter what a book or a doctor says, you know your child better than anybody else, and you really have to go by your instincts and handle your own child your own way."
- "You do learn to cope with it. You learn more about it. You always hate it, and it will always rip your heart

out that your child has it, this terrible disease. Just learn to live with it the best you can. It's not easy. You give them the shot with a 'Let's get it over with and not make a big deal out of it' although it's ripping your heart out every minute."

- "*Everyone* is handicapped in some manner. Some handicaps are visible, ones that require wheelchairs, braces, etc., or ones like obesity or chronic acne; other handicaps are not visible, like hypertension or liver disease, nearsightedness, or diabetes. It was illustrated for me that a handicap, any handicap, is just a uniqueness—something all our own. I try to share that concept with my daughter when explaining that diabetes is not something she 'is' but rather something she 'has.' I try to get across the message that she hasn't been singled out or punished by God, but that she is unique and worthwhile and that her diabetes is just a facet of all that makes her so."

- "I want other parents to realize that their children who have diabetes want to be treated as normal. They don't want attention directed toward their disease. For example, instead of ordering the diabetic meal for my son on the airline, I should have just had the regular meal served. It was not that much different, and the attention that was focused on Matt caused him much distress."

- "Any doctor who puts heavy guilt on you and tells you your child is going to die when you are trying your best should be changed to one with whom you can work realistically."

- "Tell parents to attend the latest up-to-date seminars on diabetes in their local hospitals and read the magazines put out by the ADA and JDF."

- "Get together with other parents of diabetic children and talk with them; go to support groups; get your children involved in them. Tell the parents that there's a light at the end of the tunnel for their children. One day there will be a cure. That's what keeps us going."

- "It is devastating, and it doesn't wear off. You are always fighting the clock, but the last ten years we have made great strides. We're light-years ahead with the blood glucose machine and in the research."
- "More than anything else, love your kid, but never let them feel that you love them more than you would if they didn't have diabetes. Just treat them as normally as possible, and if they're out of line, they are out of line—diabetes or no diabetes. Don't let the diabetes ever become an excuse. Sometimes that's really tough, but you've just got to keep trying to do that on a daily basis."
- "The advice that proved to be most important to me was that Matthew was a child *first*. The diabetes was something he had, but it shouldn't rule his life. The diabetes is one aspect of the total being that encompasses his mind and body. He is an artist, a runner, a mimic, a dancer, a joyful blond child, a crabby blond child, a host of things."
- "One thing that impresses me about children who have diabetes is their courage . . .

> 365 days a year
> 3 times a day—an injection
> 4 times a day—blood tests that leave little
>   fingers all pokey-looking
> Every day—the changes in mood if the blood
>   sugar rises or falls too fast

"The bumps and lumps from shots—even if you rotate the sites. The shots that you give and try not to hurt but sometimes do . . . and they have them every day!

"Now *that* bravery impresses me!"
- "I'd tell parents to never give up hope and to hug their children . . . a lot."

11
Specifics: Questions from Parents

This chapter was put together from the dozens of parent interviews I conducted. There were so many questions parents had, even after years of experience with diabetes, that I felt the answers needed to be shared with you.

Dr. Robert Clemons provided most of the medical information for this chapter. Dr. Clemons is a pediatric endocrinologist in Glendale, California. He is a fellow of the American Academy of Pediatrics, a member of the Lawson-Wilkes Pediatric Endocrine Society, a member of the American Diabetes Association, attending physician of the Division of Endocrinology at Children's Hospital of Los Angeles, and clinical associate and professor of pediatrics at the USC School of Medicine.

My 12-year-old daughter doesn't want to talk about her diabetes. She doesn't want anyone to know. I'm worried that her denial will lead to problems.

Your daughter doesn't have to talk about it or tell everyone if she doesn't wish to do that. It's her diabetes, and her right to privacy should be respected. If she is taking her blood tests and shots and taking reasonably good care of herself, she is not really denying it.

Even though she doesn't have to tell everyone, she should be encouraged to let some people who are close to her know. She might feel her diabetes is something to be ashamed of. She needs to be helped to see the other side—that good friends will respect her ability to deal with all the shots and finger pricks. Perhaps she

needs to practice how to tell friends about diabetes. It's
scary to tell people something important about
ourselves and feel they might reject us. She needs help
to understand that if no one knows, no one can help
her if she has a serious reaction. Most of all, she needs
a lot of reassurance.

Your daughter is old enough now to understand the
impact diabetes has on her life. Also, for the first time,
she is aware of what the future could hold with regard
to complications. She may be experiencing a sense of
loss, fear of the future, and may actually be somewhat
depressed. The early adolescent is also very concerned
with body image and being like everyone else. The
differentness of having diabetes can be very distressing
for some children.

If you notice that her grades are falling or she has any
other big changes in outward behavior such as weight
loss or decreased compliance, forging test results, anger,
or hostility, your daughter may need extra help. If she
won't open up to you or another adult, ask your doctor
to recommend a therapist to help her explore her
feelings.

How do I know my child is receiving the best possible care for her diabetes?

First of all, your child should be under the care of a
diabetes specialist. If possible, find a pediatric
diabetologist or endocrinologist in your area. You will
also need a diabetes educator, a nutritionist or dietitian,
and an ophthalmologist who is a retina or diabetic
retinopathy specialist. A pediatric endocrinologist may
be hard to find. If so, an adult endocrinologist or a well-
trained pediatrician who cares for a large number of
Type I diabetic patients would also be a good choice.
Diabetes is a special disease and requires the care of a
specialist.

One of the best ways to find a doctor is through
personal recommendations from people knowledgeable

about diabetes and from other doctors. Other parents of diabetics will be eager to share a good doctor with you. You can call your local Juvenile Diabetes Foundation chapter or American Diabetes Association for lists of doctors in your area.

If you can't find a specialist close to home, check with a teaching or university hospital in a nearby large city. You could use a local nurse-educator or pediatrician/family doctor in combination with a specialist so that you could call when you needed advice. The local physician or nurse-educator could provide the information and support you need for daily care, and you could make the longer trip to the specialist for checkups. Either way, a diabetes educator and a nutritionist are very helpful because even a well-trained, well-meaning physician doesn't always have the time to spend with the family or the patient to go over the fine details, particularly in the area of diet.

If your child is being treated by a doctor who is not a diabetes specialist, and diabetics do not account for a large portion of his practice, your child may not be getting the best care. If your child's doctor does not recommend blood glucose monitoring or feel it's necessary, get another opinion. Home blood glucose monitoring is the most important advance in the quality of care of diabetics since insulin was discovered. There is every good reason why your child should be using it.

You deserve a doctor who explains what the blood tests and diabetes care techniques mean. You should not be kept in the dark. You also don't need a doctor who makes you feel guilty for disturbing him with questions.

Your child's checkups should include a physical examination, a discussion of the blood-test records (which should be brought to each visit), and a special blood test called a *hemoglobin A1C* or glycosylated hemoglobin. Ideally, this test should be done every three to four months or, at least, twice a year. Your doctor or

an associate should be available to you by phone on a
24-hour basis so that significant changes in control or
illness can be tended to immediately. This is especially
important if your child is newly diagnosed. Your child
should also be examined by the ophthalmologist once a
year.

**My child is on one shot a day. Will we need to switch
to two or three injections?**

Most diabetes specialists are now recommending at
least two injections a day. For a one-shot program to be
considered successful, it should ideally provide the
following elements of control:

1. Morning glucose between 80 and 120 with
occasionally a little higher and not too often lower (a
little higher is especially desirable for the younger child
who can't report reactions as reliably).

2. Maintaining 80–150 blood sugar during the day
without reactions (100–180 for under-school-age
children).

The problem is that, as the insulin dose increases,
only one shot makes it more difficult to give enough
NPH to carry through the nighttime. Two shots a day
allow more flexible control. Recommendations for three
and four shots are becoming more common, allowing
even greater flexibility and control.

Do you have any tricks for giving painless injections?

The only real trick is to use the smallest-gauge needle
(like a 27-gauge microfine needle) and insert it quickly,
either with a quick stabbing motion or a flip-of-the-
wrist motion. The discomfort of a shot comes from two
things: the needle going through the skin (hence thin,
sharp needles inserted *quickly*) and the spreading of
tissues by the fluid that's being injected. To avoid pain
here, the insulin should be injected *slowly*.

The atmosphere surrounding shot time can help too. First of all, try to calm yourself if you are anxious. Take a few deep breaths, think loving, happy thoughts, say a little prayer, whatever helps you to relax. Choose a comfortable, peaceful place, a sofa or chair in a quiet part of the house. Distracting a child by talking about the pleasant things that will happen after the shot is over can help, too. Brennan occasionally used to get very anxious about his shots, even after the first few years. Just at the moment I inserted the needle, my housekeeper would call to him and ask him about something he liked or wanted. Most of the time, it helped. Physical distraction is especially good for younger children. Give them something fascinating to play with or examine.

Try not to give a shot in the midst of an argument. Also, don't negotiate with your child over whether or not the shot will be given. It will, and there's no choice. Try not to delay the shot. Putting off the difficult doesn't make it less difficult. Do give your child whatever choices you can. For example, let her select the injection site. Be sure to end with a big hug.

(As I write these instructions, I remember days when we had to hold Brennan down in order to give him his shot. I don't think anything has ever been more painful than hearing him say, "Mommy, don't," and having to do it anyway. It's so easy to write the words and give advice or instructions. Some days it's so hard to follow them.)

Most health professionals will recommend that disposable needles be used only once and then discarded. Many parents do reuse syringes to save money. Several parents I interviewed reported that reusing them presented no problem. After two usages, the needle may become dull. Be sure to recap the needle immediately after use and never reuse syringes with bent or dirty needles.

Does it help or hinder my child to discuss with him the fact that good control will affect his long-term well-being?

Of course, up to a certain age, probably late childhood or the early teens, such a discussion will not be fully comprehensible to the child. I think it all depends on when and how it is presented. In all cases, it should be done in a caring, sensitive manner. Such discussion can inflict fear of the long-term consequences and create guilt for the child, especially if he's not complying as well as he feels he should. However, it is crucial, as the child gets older and becomes more responsible for his actions, that he clearly understands that what he does will have an effect on his diabetes in the long run.

I remember a young woman who was 27 years old and was losing her sight after having had diabetes for 15 years. She said no one ever told her that there were long-term consequences of bad control. During her teens, she rebelled against her diabetes and refused to care for herself. Her mother and doctor admonished and nagged her but never told her the whole story of what diabetes can do. She feels that if she had known what could happen, she probably would have been more careful.

I am not recommending threatening your child into living up to ideal standards of control. That can often backfire. But even if you don't directly mention complications, your child may hear about them. People will say, "You have diabetes? That's awful. My father died of diabetes," or "My aunt went blind from diabetes." You'll need to deal with your child's feelings about that. Keep your explanation as general and nonthreatening as possible. Something like "Diabetes can hurt some people if they don't take good care of themselves" is best. Give honest, straightforward information to the questions you are asked. If a child senses that something is being hidden, his fears may be

worse than his reality. Be sure to stress the immediate
positive rewards of controlling diabetes—feeling good,
growing well, and staying out of the hospital.

**People on the outside have no concept that diabetes
isn't like the sniffles. It's a 24-hour, 7-day-a-week job.
We need something to give us all some inner strength
or self-esteem to face the insensitivity that really is
out there in the world. We don't want to create barriers
between ourselves and the outside world but to be able
to insulate ourselves to the insensitivity.**

There is no way to insulate or isolate yourself from what
other people say and do, but there are some things you
can do to make life with diabetes easier.

First of all, align yourself with other parents who are
doing something positive about diabetes. Don't just
accept it as fate; fight it! Your child's life and well-being
are challenged by diabetes. Become a parent-advocate,
an emissary, an educator. Remember that it wasn't too
long ago that you knew nothing about diabetes.
Insensitivity is often born of ignorance. You have a
chance to change that ignorance. Don't shy away from
it. Take on the responsibility of being a public relations
expert on behalf of diabetes and your child. It will help
you feel less a victim of diabetes if you take control.

Your self-esteem need not be in jeopardy. You and your
family have been handed a chronic illness. If you take
responsibility for it and learn all you can, you should
feel a sense of accomplishment for your achievement.

The barriers that exist are all abstract—emotional or
psychological—and they can be overcome. For example,
you may find that some former friends avoid you. They
may do that because they don't know what to do or say.
The burden falls on you to reach out, to be assertive, to
educate. You need to look like you're handling it. If you
look miserable, people are going to stay away. You need
to help them feel comfortable about asking questions.

The more you reach out and educate and share what

you know and feel, the stronger you'll be, not just for
yourself but for your child. One of the steps of the
program of Alcoholics Anonymous (another chronic
illness) asks the alcoholic to share the program with
others, to reach out. Like love, the more you give, the
more you have. That goes for diabetes too.

**We haven't been away from our child since she was
diagnosed. We need a break, but we're afraid to leave
her with anyone else.**

This is a very common reaction for parents, especially
with younger diabetics. You're right; you do need a
break. If you've gotten involved in JDF, or an ADA
support group, you've met other parents like you. Ask if
you could give them a night off by looking after their
child if they'll do the same for you. Even one night away
can feel like a whole vacation. If your child is under
good control and the caretaker is properly educated,
everything will probably go so smoothly that you'll feel
disappointed that you're so easily expendable. If no
family member or other parent can be found, you might
consider having a nurse come in, just to give the shot.
By the way, almost anyone can learn to give a shot. The
toughest part is making sure the dosage is correct.
Until Brennan began giving his own shot, every
housekeeper and secretary I've had learned to give
injections. We never had a mishap. You might be able to
find diabetic teens who will baby-sit through your
doctor, educator, or support group.

   If all else fails and there's no one to give the shots, go
out just after your child's evening shot. You and your
spouse can also arrange to give each other a night out
with friends.

**My child is still young, and I've been able to keep all
undesirable foods away from him so far. I worry about
how much longer I can do that.**

Well, you must realize it can't go on forever. You can't

protect your child from undesirable foods. Support good health habits in your own home and educate your child about good nutrition. Steer him toward healthier treats and tell him why. Work an occasional dessert into his diet plan. Get him active in sports so that he sees the relationship between exercise and blood sugar control. One of anything is not a disaster if day-to-day control is reasonably good. Learn how to adjust insulin dosages and figure exchanges and teach your child. Give him the flexibility to adapt diabetes to his life within healthy guidelines. Give him the chance to make choices. Let him know there are alternatives to the treats his friends eat that taste good and fit his diet. Help him have the strength and courage to do what he needs to do.

How do I deal with my diabetic child's awareness of her own mortality? Nicole will mention occasionally her concern that she might die. It is always confusing and upsetting for me. No matter how I deal with it, I often wonder if I'm handling it the right way.

There are several important elements to consider when forming your answer. Up to the age of 6, a child's prevelant fear is of separation. From 6 to 11, pain and death are of great concern. Listen to the way your child formulates the question. If she's worried that diabetes may cause her death, you need to tell the truth but in a very nonthreatening, positive way. For example, "Diabetes is a disease that some people can die from, especially if they've had it for a very long time, but you're doing very well, and that's why it's important to take good care of yourself." Try to understand what your child's needs are at the moment. If she's merely asking a general question about death, don't inject your own fears into the conversation or answer what you're afraid she might be asking. If you're not sure what she's asking, help her be more specific. Answer the exact question your child asks. Don't go into detailed

description if it's not needed. Build a base of
information and expand it as she gets older and her
questions become more specific.

How can my child go to bed with a normal blood sugar and wake up high?

The most common causes of elevated early morning
blood sugar are inadequate nighttime NPH and too
much food for the bedtime snack. Gradually increasing
the dose of NPH at dinnertime and performing morning
glucose readings will help the first problem. Work with
your doctor and/or dietitian on changes for the bedtime
snack.

Be aware that, from time to time, all diabetic children
will sneak extra food or will be eating more food than is
allotted in their diet. Obviously, excess calorie intake,
especially if the food is taken without the parents'
knowledge, is another reason for elevated blood glucoses
in the morning.

Another possible cause is that your child is having
low blood sugars in the middle of the night, and, in
response to the hypoglycemia, is having early morning
elevated blood sugars. You can check this by waking
your child during the night at various times and testing
her blood. If she is getting too low, it may mean that she
has too much NPH in her evening dose and that either
that dosage should be lowered or her bedtime snack
should be increased.

Finally, if none of the above apply, it could possibly be
something called the "dawn phenomenon." The dawn
phenomenon is not completely understood yet, but it is
the occurrence of an early morning (usually 4:00 to 6:00
A.M.) rise in blood sugar. The currently accepted
explanation is that this rise is due to a combination of
factors. We know that the blood cortisone levels rise
gradually during the night to a peak level at
approximately 8:00 A.M. Cortisone can cause a definite
increase in sugar output from the liver and is felt to be

in part responsible for the dawn phenomenon. In addition, growth hormone, which is manufactured in the pituitary gland, is released during sleep. It is known that growth hormone can decrease the uptake of glucose into the tissues and thus also contribute to an elevated blood sugar. If your child does seem to be experiencing a high morning blood sugar due to the dawn phenomenon, your doctor may recommend that you begin a three-shot program. Children on this program usually take regular and NPH before breakfast and then take just regular insulin before dinner. The third shot would be an injection of NPH given at bedtime so that its peak action comes later during the night, at the time when the blood sugar is rising. Many times, this increased insulin activity in the early morning hours will counteract the tendency toward rising blood sugar at the time and allow the child to achieve better early morning control.

I want to add a footnote about blood sugar control in general. The endocrine system is very complex, and the hormones are powerful stimuli in the body. Poor control may alter the hormone levels to a point where the liver is stimulated to pour out large amounts of sugar, creating even worse control. Getting a diabetic in good control may lead to normalization of the hormones involved and to a decrease in the output of glucose from the liver. So good control may actually cause your child to be in better control. What a nice bonus!

What happens when my child is ill? Also, please explain ketoacidosis.

Illness is always a kind of a compromise between eating less, which decreases insulin requirements, and the sickness and fever, which increase insulin requirements. Illness has been shown to increase the glucagon output from the liver. Glucagon is a protein hormone. It is made in the alpha cells of the pancreas, right next to the beta cells that produce insulin.

Glucagon has effects opposite those of insulin; it is actually a blood sugar raiser. It works by causing the liver to release glucose. Increased glucagon may cause increased glucose output from the liver and cause an actual increased need for insulin. Fever increases the rate of metabolism and insulin need as well. So a child with a cold or an illness that isn't affecting his ability to eat probably has increased insulin needs. A child with an illness that affects her ability to eat and take in food is in a conflict between the increased insulin needs of illness and the decreased insulin needs from lowered food intake. The insulin doses sometimes have to be decreased or perhaps maintained at the same level even though a child is not able to eat, in order to keep them in control. Then, of course, if the child is vomiting, she's losing body fluids. The vomiting and the fever may just make it easier for the whole cycle of ketoacidosis to get started and to progress. The patient who is in borderline control can slip into ketoacidosis more easily, because his hormonal system may already be out of balance.

Ketoacidosis usually begins with insulin deficiency. The first thing that happens with insulin deficiency is an elevation of blood sugar (since sugar is unable to get into the tissues without insulin). Then, as the blood sugar gets higher, the level of sugar exceeds the level at which the kidney can keep it all inside. Sugar then spills into the urine, and as the level of sugar gets greater, it pulls more and more water with it, and there is an increase in the volume of urination. This increased urination causes fluid loss from the body. Since the body is losing extra fluid, another consequence of this fluid loss is increased thirst. Increased urine volume and increased thirst are the early warning signs that your child is getting out of control and that you need to take action.

At the same time as the above changes are taking place, the cells sense a lack of sugar because of the lack of insulin. Hormone changes in the body start to take place, causing the liver to put out more sugar and adding to the high blood sugar levels. The body also begins to break down fats to use as energy since it can't use its normal fuel, glucose. As the body begins to burn these fats, the bloods becomes more acidic, and ketones or acetone accumulates in the blood. (The ketones or acetone are by-products of the breakdown of fats.) As the acidity of the blood increases due to fat breakdown, the body tries to compensate for this acidity by causing at first deep and then more rapid respirations. The child who has significant ketoacidosis may actually look as if he is out of breath from running. Simultaneously, abdominal pains and discomfort can occur, and the child becomes nauseated and begins to vomit. Once the child begins to vomit, and is, therefore, unable to drink and replace the increased body fluids lost in the urine, he begins to become more dehydrated. If this process continues, the child can rapidly slip into diabetic coma, a condition which can be life threatening if not treated promptly.

One key point is that *everybody needs to have insulin every day.* Even if you taped your child's mouth shut, she'd need insulin. The pitfalls people fall into are "I didn't give her insulin because she was vomiting," and "I thought if she didn't eat she didn't need insulin." In reality, you need insulin from minute to minute to run your body. The body's prime fuel is glucose, and it can't get into the cells without insulin. So your insulin requirement is made up of two basic elements: the amount of insulin you need just to keep your body going and an additional amount of insulin necessary to metabolize the food that you do eat.

What this means to a parent of a diabetic child is that any illness necessitates watchfulness. You need to test your child's blood more frequently, perhaps even every one to two hours. Urine testing also is important. Check for urine spillage and presence of ketones. Your doctor may also ask you to keep track of urine volume. A diabetic child can go from moderately ill to seriously ill in a very short time. If your child's blood sugar is over 400, and the urine shows large ketones, call your doctor. If the doctor cannot be reached, get your child to a hospital immediately. Keep in close touch with your doctor during illness. Have your doctor or nurse-educator call the hospital and pave the way at the emergency room. At least call the hospital yourself and let them know you're on your way, and see who's on call. You want to be sure whoever treats your child knows something about diabetes and ketoacidosis. I've heard stories of children with ketoacidosis who were put on a glucose IV.

Your child will need to ingest 35 to 50 grams of carbohydrate every four hours during illness. Twelve ounces of regular (nondiet) soft drink, orange juice, or tea sweetened with 3 tablespoons of sugar would provide 30 grams of carbohydrate. For a younger child, 30 grams would probably be sufficient. A child over the age of 10 to 12 years would need closer to 50 grams. These amounts are approximate guidelines. Your doctor will provide precise recommendations for your child based on the total picture of insulin intake, blood sugar, etc.

What do I do when my daughter calls from school saying she doesn't feel well and I'm left with the suspicion that there's a math test that day? I'm sure I've been a chump on many occasions.

There are ways to avoid being a chump. Lots of kids with and without diabetes try the "I don't feel very well" on test-day trick. If your daughter has blood-testing equipment at school, have her test and, if she's low, eat a proper snack to bring the blood sugar back to normal. If there's no blood-testing equipment at school, offer to drive over and test her. You can ask her if she's absolutely sure her diabetes is causing a problem. If not, and there are no other symptoms of illness like fever, ask her to be very specific about what's bothering her and deal with it as you would any nondiabetic child. A slightly elevated blood sugar is not an excuse to miss school. Some children will try to use their diabetes to manipulate their parents. Discuss guidelines for keeping your child home from school with your child's doctor.

Please give me information on insulin reactions, how to avoid them, how to handle them, whether they are dangerous, etc.

Insulin reactions occur when there is more insulin than food (glucose). The blood sugar drops below a normal low-end level (60–70), and the child starts to display symptoms. There are so many factors that affect blood sugar—insulin dosage, food intake, exercise, stress, weather, and even altitude. The best way to avoid low blood sugar is through experience, watchfulness, and overall good control. You learn what affects your child's blood sugar by observation. Also be aware that during the summer months or on special outings, your child's activity level may change significantly. You may need to compensate for the increased activity by lowering the insulin dose and/or increasing food intake.

In regard to insulin dosage, if your child has a pattern of reactions in mid-morning or two to three hours after his breakfast shot, his regular insulin is peaking and he needs either less insulin or more food. Juice or any other simple carbohydrate will bring the blood sugar back to normal and can be followed by a protein and carbohydrate such as cheese and crackers. Also, be sure your child always has a source of glucose with her and is educated to know how to handle reactions when she is not with you.

It is easy to "overfeed" an insulin reaction. During an insulin reaction, the body's own hormone responses attempt to raise blood sugar by causing sugar release from the liver and even manufacturing new sugar from protein in the liver. If large amounts of sugared foods are given at a time when the body is also trying to raise its own sugar levels, excess elevation of blood sugar can occur, and that's not desirable either! Remember that it takes 10 to 20 minutes for a reaction to subside. If your child isn't feeling better in 20 minutes, check his blood sugar again, and, if he's still low, give him more sugar and food. Discuss the parameters of feeding a reaction with your dietitian or doctor.

If the reactions occur more than four to six hours after a shot, it is probably the NPH or Lente insulin that is responsible (if a pattern of reactions is established). Then the NPH or Lente should be reduced. Reduction should continue on a daily basis until a normal blood sugar pattern is reestablished. One or two units may be all that is necessary for a child under five.

If your child is suffering reactions (as a pattern) in the middle of the night, the NPH is the culprit. You'll need to lower the dinner NPH or increase the bedtime snack. You may find, as some families have, that a third shot of NPH just before bedtime will do the trick (along with eliminating the NPH at supper). That way, the NPH given at 10:00 P.M. will be peaking between 6:00 and 8:00 A.M. instead of between 2:00 and 4:00 A.M. There'll be less chance of reactions in the wee hours and more likelihood of good morning readings.

Exercise burns glucose. It makes insulin more effective. So, extra exercise means extra food. You need to be aware of the time an insulin will peak and the time the additional exercise will take place. For example, a soccer game at 3:00 in the afternoon means your child's NPH will be peaking. Soccer is a very physically demanding game. In addition to an extra snack, you might want to consider giving your child a little less NPH in the morning shot. Also, three to four hours of strenuous exercise may lower insulin needs for eight to 16 hours. For example, beware of morning

reactions the night after a bike-a-thon. Discuss it with
your doctor.

There are four basic names for insulin. Here's a little
chart that may help you identify each one and its
action:

	Starts Working	Peaks	Lasts
Regular (rapid-acting)	30 minutes–1 hour	2–4 hours	6–8 hours
NPH (intermediate)	2–4 hours	6–10 hours	12–24 hours
Lente (intermediate)	2–4 hours	6–10 hours	12–24 hours
Ultralente (long-acting)	3–4 hours	DOESN'T	24–36 hours

Most diabetic children are on a two- to three-shot
program using regular and NPH or Lente. Ultralente can
be a problem for some people because it stays active for
over 24 hours. This can sometimes lead to an insulin
reaction when the Ultralente hasn't worn off and the
new breakfast shot has started working. Ultralente is
also formulated with beef insulin, which for some
people can cause insulin resistance. Pork and human
insulin are more like a person's own insulin and rarely
cause those problems.

Knowing how each insulin works will help you
understand the possible causes when a reaction takes
place.

Stress (good and bad) can affect blood sugar because
the hormonal system is affected by stress. For example,
the night before his grandfather's funeral, one young
boy had a severe reaction. Another teenage girl could
feel her blood sugar rising as a handsome new student
joined her class. She excused herself and tested her
blood. She was over 400!

Sometimes the reactions can get really severe. It may
never happen to your child, but I want you to know
what happens when your child has a convulsion and
what to do.

When Brennan was diagnosed, there was so much to
grasp that I didn't really understand what the doctor

meant when he said that if Brennan lost consciousness,
I should give him the glucagon. I thought he would just
be very drowsy or look like he was asleep. What did
happen was a nightmare.

Brennan's father was out of town and he was
sleeping in bed with me. We had overslept a little, and I
suddenly felt the bed shaking. I thought it was an
earthquake. I got out of bed and realized the floor
wasn't shaking. I turned and looked back and saw
Brennan. His body was rigid, his eyes rolled back, and
his body was jerking violently. Blood was coming from
his mouth. (His locked jaw had pushed a loose tooth out
of its socket.) Sugar! I ran to the kitchen and could find
only packets of sugar. I realized he couldn't swallow
anything. Then I remembered the glucagon. I got it and
ran to the phone. Meanwhile, my girlfriend, who had
stayed over, was in with Brennan. I got the doctor on
the line, and she led me through the procedure of
loading the glucagon. My hands were shaking so badly I
got only half of it loaded, but she said that was enough.
I injected it into his abdomen, and within minutes he
came around.

Before that day, I had not been able to get Brennan to
do a blood test without a struggle. We would have to
hold him down. The anger and rage that came out of
him was a terrible thing to see as a parent. We had
decided to put off blood-testing for a while until
Brennan could handle it better.

Immediately after the convulsion, he was a little
dazed, and I was able to get the blood tests done. Even
after the glucagon, his test was only about 60. Then he
started throwing up. Glucagon can upset the stomach.
We had quite a time trying to keep liquids in him and
keeping his blood sugar normal that day.

Don't be caught unaware as I was. Your child can
have a convulsion, and you should be prepared. Have
your doctor or diabetes educator take you through a dry
run of loading the glucagon. The practice will be

important if an emergency should arise. Always have cake frosting in a tube and/or glucagon handy wherever your child is. The cake frosting can be squeezed between the cheek and teeth and will be absorbed quickly. Ask your doctor for additional methods of dealing with a convulsion.

The best way to avoid severe reactions is to have your child under good control. Convulsions can be harmful, so take the possibility of them seriously and be prepared.

What is good control, and can you give any tricks of the trade for achieving better control?

Many times, if our child has a close to normal blood sugar before his shots, we feel the control is good. There's another element to consider. It's called the *post-prandial blood sugar*. Post-prandial means after eating. Your child's post-prandial blood sugar tells us how well the insulin is covering the carbohydrate in his meal. In addition to checking the blood sugar prior to insulin injections, you should also check sugars two hours after meals, before lunch, and at bedtime on a rotating basis to see that the blood sugar remains within acceptable limits throughout the day rather than just prior to shots.

Good control or tight control should mimic the body's natural response to eating. The body always has some insulin present in the system and then adds more insulin, exactly measured to fit the amount of food ingested. That's why we give our children long-acting (NPH or Lente) and short-acting (regular) insulin. No two days are exactly alike for a diabetic child in terms of food, exercise, and stress. That's why adjusting the insulin dosage and/or waiting between shots and meals help to imitate the nondiabetic's body. The regular insulin can be adjusted on a daily basis with the NPH being adjusted more slowly after trends in blood sugar are ascertained. Your doctor or educator can advise you on this. As time goes by, you will come to know what to do even better than your doctor. You are with your child 24 hours a day. Your doctor doesn't live in your pocket and can't possibly know your child's body and its daily fluctuations as well as you do. Eventually, you and your child will gain confidence in adjusting insulin, food intake, or waiting time to respond to the blood tests.

The goal for teenagers should be a blood sugar range of 80 to 150 before breakfast or anytime food is not eaten for two hours. Younger school-age children might aim for 80 to 180. Preschool children should be kept in the range of 100 to 180, if possible. These are goals to work toward.

It's important to remember that these are ideal goals. Don't have unrealistic expectations or blame your child if his blood sugar is out of control. One high blood sugar is not a disaster. Work together to figure out what might have caused the higher than usual blood sugar.

The hemoglobin A1C or glycosolated hemoglobin is another valuable tool your doctor uses to judge control. It measures the amount of glucose that clings to the hemoglobin (the red substance in our blood that carries oxygen to the tissues). The higher the average blood sugar level, the higher the glycosolated hemoglobin level will be. Since the blood cells containing the hemoglobin live about 120 days, changes in the glycosolated hemoglobin level are very slow (unlike the blood sugar levels, which change from minute to minute) and can give an indication of how a patient's overall control has been over the last several months.

One mother whose daughter's before-meal tests were near normal found that the Hemoglobin A1C showed a different picture. It turned out that her daughter's post-prandial sugar was high. By waiting between shots and meals and spot-checking after meals, she was able to bring her daughter under much better control.

There are rewards for good control. First, on an immediate level, your child feels good and has fewer reactions. Second, there are many indications that tight control may help your child delay or avoid complications. For parents, that's a priority.

You need to give the regular insulin time to start working before you put more glucose into the body. There's a system of waiting times you can use. Use this information as a rough rule of thumb and tailor the waiting times to your own child, based on post-prandial blood sugar tests. If those tests are close to normal, but your child is having reactions an hour or so later, the control may be too tight and you should adjust accordingly.

- With tests between 120 and 170, wait 30 minutes.
- With tests between 170 and 200, wait at least 45 minutes. With Brennan, we wait 60 minutes or more, and he doesn't show signs of reaction.
- With tests between 200 and 240, wait 60 minutes.

The waiting time is a valuable tool for better control. We use it now instead of adding more regular insulin, when Brennan is higher than he should be. The hemoglobin A1C and spot-check blood tests will give testimony to how well it's working. For some families, especially in the morning when schedules can be hectic, waiting one hour between the insulin injection and breakfast may not be possible. At this time, instead of increasing the time between insulin injection and food intake, a sliding scale of insulin dose adjustment can be given to you by your physician so you know that for a given blood sugar, you need to add a certain number of units of regular insulin to compensate for the higher blood sugar. Discuss it with your doctor or educator.

I worry about my other children resenting the time and attention I give my diabetic child.

Diabetes creates a lot of extra work and worries for a parent. There's extra time and planning involved in

caring for a diabetic, and other siblings can get jealous.
It can manifest itself as regressive behavior. Rather
than treat babyish behavior by the Joan Rivers method
("Oh, grow up!"), use hugs and extra attention to
placate the regressive party. We all need extra babying
now and then. Plan a small outing with that sibling.
Even a shopping trip together because "I really need
your help" can be effective. Let your child overhear you
telling someone else how good she is at _____.
Acknowledge all that is done well every chance you get.
Your other child needs to know she is important, too.
Sometimes siblings are afraid that they too will get
diabetes. Reassure them that the odds are low.

I remember when Robin, my younger son, was four, he
said to me, "Brennan has diabetes. What do I have?" I
told him he had cute buns. He smiled and seemed
pleased by that answer.

Look on the bright side. The extra time you spend
with your diabetic child and then with other siblings in
compensating for the time you spend with your diabetic
creates lots of family togetherness! As one father said, "I
never knew Walt Disney made so many movies."

Sometimes your other children don't understand the
seriousness of diabetes until they see what a bad
reaction can be like. Several families I interviewed
reported a definite change in siblings' attitudes after
such an incident. Be sure siblings know how to handle
a reaction, give glucagon, how they can help. Let them
know how important their help is.

All through this book, I have tried to convince you of
the many benefits of your family's following the basic
diabetic way of eating. This doesn't mean you should
expect siblings to follow a diet as strict as your diabetic
child. While it's unfair to leave candy lying around the
house, it's also unnatural to let a child expect that the
whole world revolves around his diabetes. Every child
with diabetes must learn to exist in the real world. If
your other children are having a treat, provide an

appropriate choice for your diabetic child. Or you can plan a special dessert when your diabetic child is out of the house, sleeping, or having a nap. If other family members know they can have their favorite disgustingly gooey dessert once in a while, the resentment will be considerably less. It's not sneaking; it's just being sensitive to your diabetic child's feelings. One more word about forbidden foods. Give your child the knowledge with which to "cheat" without hurting himself and there'll be less sneaking around.

Could you give me some tips for being organized enough to handle any diabetes emergency?

Have a booklet or loose-leaf notebook that outlines your child's diet, insulin dosages, symptoms of reactions, and treatments, along with doctors' phone numbers. One mother called her book "The Care and Feeding of Bradley." Also, always have extra supplies handy for blood tests and food and glucose sources for reactions. A basket in the car and one in the kitchen filled with cake frosting in a tube, cans of juice, and packages of cheese and crackers will come in handy and are easy to pick up and take with you at a moment's notice. Have a zippered case for the insulin syringes and testing equipment. There are several available that are specially designed for diabetes supplies. They are advertised in the ADA magazine, *Diabetes Forecast.* We use a man's dop kit or shaving kit imprinted with Brennan's initials. Once again, include all family members in planning for emergencies.

Will a therapist be able to get my teenager to stick to his diet?

A parent's and doctor's fantasy may be that a therapist will make the child comply. Compliance, per se, is not the role of the therapist. If the therapist lectures and takes the stance of another authority figure who tries to control, he will lose the child. The goal of the therapist is to provide a time for the child to talk about what's on his mind and help reduce stress. Compliance may follow, but of the child's own volition. When he was eight years old, Brennan wrote me a note. It said, "Life is hard. I don't want to live anymore." He didn't want to talk about it. I took him to a psychologist who had extensive experience with children with chronic illness. It took him a long time to open up, but he did change and become much more willing to talk about his feelings.

Children with chronic illness sometimes cease to trust the adults around them. We tell them we're going to help them feel better, and then we hurt them—with needles, finger pricks. For children, the major stress of diabetes is often the pain.

If possible, find a therapist familiar with diabetes. Inquire through your hospital's department of social work or psychology. If your therapist doesn't know about diabetes, help educate him by supplying him with reading material.

I worry that the diet sodas we're served in restaurants may not always be sugar-free.

Just as urine strips will indicate sugar in the urine, they'll also indicate sugar in a soft drink. You can carry some with your child's supplies and use them whenever you're unsure. For "professional" advice on diet versus nondiet drinks, we ask my son Robin. He hates diet sodas and can identify a sugar-free soda at 50 paces!

I'm worried about alcohol and my teenaged diabetic. Any advice?

Well, once again, you can give information and advice and hope that your teen pays attention and takes it seriously. Here are the points to make.

1. Alcohol is a rich source of calories with almost no nutrient value.
2. Alcohol behaves like fat in the body.

3. Alcohol is broken down in the liver. While the liver is processing the alcohol, it is prevented from making sugar. If the blood sugar drops below normal, the liver is not able to release glucose to counteract the insulin reaction. The danger then is twofold. Sometimes people forget to eat if they're drinking, which for a diabetic means an insulin reaction. Secondly, the reaction can be even more severe if the liver doesn't release any glucose to help.

4. If your teen is determined to have a drink now and then, ask him to drink only in moderation and only when he's already eaten. Even a glass of milk will help protect the stomach and the brain.

5. Let him know that, if he has a severe reaction while drinking, people will think he's drunk and most likely will leave him alone. An unattended insulin reaction can be dangerous and cause brain damage. Someone with him should know he has diabetes and know what to do in case of an insulin reaction. He should also wear a Medic-Alert bracelet or medallion. Have your doctor discuss this with your teen. Most important of all, set an example for your child by the manner in which you use alcohol. Use it sparingly and respectfully if at all. It's difficult to get your teen to abstain completely if you drink.

6. Let your teen know he does not need to drink to be a part of the gang. He might offer himself as the DD—Designated Driver.

I'm worried about insurance for my child. Can you give me some information?

Today's diabetic suffers the consequences of "uninsurability." All too often, people with diabetes (1) have trouble getting any health insurance, (2) have to pay very large premiums for their coverage, and (3) have trouble getting their insurers to pay for important expenses.

I'd like to share with you the discoveries I've made, which may help to prepare you in your search for an insurance plan that will best suit you and your diabetic child.

To begin with, there are two major categories of health insurance: group and individual. Of the two, group insurance is by far the least expensive and usually the easiest to get. Group policies offered through work tend to be open to all employees, regardless of their medical condition. Dependents are also likely to benefit from the same eligibility requirements. It is strongly recommended that *both* parents carry family plans if at all possible. If your child is covered under your plan, great. But as soon as you know he will be losing that coverage (marriage, college), begin researching new insurance options. It is crucial that the child make plans for finding new insurance *before* losing your plan's coverage.

Do you know the type of coverage you have? Have you ever sat down and read your policy all the way through? By taking a moment to do so now, you may save yourself a lot of headaches and frustration in the future. Here is a checklist of some of the key elements you should look for:

How many deductibles do you have?
What is the copayment of your plan?
What is the stop/loss limit?
Does your policy have a maximum benefit clause for a particular illness?
Or a maximum benefit per condition?
Is there a preexisting-condition clause?
Can family members be added to the plan at any time?
What medical supplies are covered (insulin, oral medications, syringes, and blood-and-urine-testing equipment)?
Can the plan be changed from group to individual health insurance if you leave

your job, and how is the dependent's
coverage affected by that change?

Is there a price ceiling for treatment of the
illness?

Are the payment limits in step with current
prices? (Call local hospitals for rates.)

How long a hospital stay will your basic
policy cover?

Does the company reserve the right to cancel
you/your dependent if he/she becomes a
high-risk case?

And, of utmost importance, look for a
guaranteed renewable or noncancelable
policy—if and when you convert from
group to individual coverage (during a
lapse in employment), this clause allows
the company to change the premium as it
does with all policies, but it cannot cancel
the policy.

Once reviewing your policy, if you find it does not
offer everything you would like, check with your
company's personnel office. Many companies offer more
than one choice of health insurance coverage. If yours
does, it probably also has an open enrollment period at
a specific time each year when employees can switch
from one plan to another if they wish. Research your
options and switch when you can. At the other end of
the spectrum, if you are an independent businessperson
or an employee of a business that is too small to carry
group coverage, you'll need to look elsewhere for help. If
at all possible, join a fraternal organization that offers
its members group insurance. If you are a college
graduate, check with that school's alumni association. If
you are a member of a large business or social club that
doesn't offer group coverage, contact your local
insurance company and see what steps could be taken
to offer insurance through your organization. Be
creative; investigate your options.

There is a bureau in Boston called the Medical Information Bureau that retains information on all claims paid and all applications denied. Once an application has been denied, it is filed. Many insurance companies simply check the bureau to see if a person is listed in their files as having had an application denied and then automatically deny the application request. Anyone can write to obtain information in the bureau's files: Disclosure Office, PO Box 105, Essex Station, Boston, MA 02112. (Medical information must be sent to a physician.) If you have reason to doubt whether your insurance application will be accepted, file a trial application. To do so, at the top of the application form write "Trial Application—Make No Record Unless Accepted." This will keep the information from being passed on to the bureau if it is rejected.

As a rule, when looking for an individual policy, the diabetic must consider how to make himself appear to be less of a risk to the insurance company. This is supported by documented proof of medical status. Diabetics should include results of a glycosylated hemoglobin test (A1C) with their application. This will show their control of the diabetes over a several-month period, and this, added to support from their physician, will aid their case in being accepted for insurance coverage. Remember: to insure the swiftest processing of the application, supply as much precise information about the diabetic's medical history as possible.

If your application is turned down and the diabetes is in good control, you can:

- appeal your case in writing to the insurance company.
- send a copy of your appeal to the insurance commissioner in the state where the insurance company is licensed.
- send a copy of your appeal to your congressman.

However, if you appeal a turned-down application, be prepared for a long, frustrating fight. And *do not* put your insurance search on hold in the meantime.

What if you can't find group or individual insurance? Let's explore the options. The first is pooled-risk insurance. These plans are intended for persons who are not eligible for group health insurance, Medicare, or Medicaid and who cannot obtain adequate health insurance in the private marketplace. The insured must be state residents who have been rejected or canceled by two or more health insurers.

These plans are currently available in eight states: Rhode Island, Minnesota, Nebraska, Connecticut, Florida, Indiana, North Dakota, and Wisconsin. States considering pooled-risk insurance are California, Mississippi, Missouri, and Ohio.

Every state plan, except Rhode Island's, requires payment of a health insurance premium with the rate ranging from 125 to 200 percent of the standard individual premium rate. As with any insurance plan, premiums vary depending on the applicant's condition.

If your state does not offer pooled-risk insurance, contact your state representatives and talk to them about sponsoring a bill providing for this plan. Another great resource will be the American Diabetes Association, which has done a lot of work in this area. This is a good way to find others in your area who are interested in helping you get this legislation going.

If you want to learn more about shared-risk plans, contact the state Department of Insurance in the states that currently have plans. A model bill for pooled-risk legislation can be obtained by writing to the National Association of Insurance Commissioners, 1125 Grand Street, Kansas City, MO 64106.

There's another alternative offered by a select group of hospitals: The Hill-Burton Act, established by Congress in 1946, provides certain hospitals and medical facilities with funds for construction and rehabilitation. The institutions that received the funds agreed to provide services for patients who could not pay. To determine which hospitals in your area

participate in the program, and whether or not you
qualify, phone 800-638-0742.

Another option here is Health Maintenance
Organizations (HMOs). For a fixed fee, you get a wide
range of medical services; regardless of the care you
may require from the HMO, you pay only the fee, no
more, no less. An HMO may be located in one building
staffed by doctors and health professionals, or it may be
served by professionals working out of their own offices.
Major health problems are handled by hospitals
connected with the HMO. The positive side of HMOs is
that they tend to emphasize prevention. The negative
side is that you are limited to using only doctors and
facilities connected with the HMO. If you want to see a
diabetes specialist and there is none on the HMO's
staff, you'll have to pay to see one yourself.

An all too common problem is that people just don't
know what kind of coverage they have until it's too late
to do anything about it. Read your policy and
investigate the options. If you are going to change jobs
and plan to convert your coverage from group to
individual, check on the conversion privilege and the
amount of time you have to convert that policy. *Don't
wait until the last minute.* Losing your established
coverage can be disastrous, forcing you to have to prove
your dependent's insurability—and for a diabetic, that's
where the problem lies.

The following is a recent list of insurers you may
contact for further information.

Diabetes Group Insurance Trust Plans
c/o Jon W. Hall & Associates Inc.
PO Box 14868
Shawnee Mission, KS 66215
(913) 268-7878 or (800) 527-0965

Diabetic Insurance Programs
PO Box 72
Westport, CT 06881
Call collect: (203) 226-9911

Harold Bresnick & Associates
230 Park Ave.
New York, NY 10169
(212) 697-9884

Department of Social Security for Federal Aid
(SSI)

Crippled Children's Associations on the state
level, as well as Vocational Rehabilitation

12
Resources

This chapter is meant to assist you in finding support and information concerning diabetes. It is a partial list of resources available based on sources that I have actually used or that have been recommended to me. There are two major sources of help and hope for people with diabetes in North America. They are the American Diabetes Association (and the Canadian Diabetes Association) and the Juvenile Diabetes Foundation International. You should join both for a variety of reasons.

ADA AND JDF

The ADA is a great source of diabetes education, both for professionals and for diabetics and their families. The ADA magazine, *Diabetes Forecast*, is, I feel, must reading for any family struggling with this disease. It is filled with articles on the physical, emotional, and psychological aspects of diabetes as well as updates on the latest research, lobbying efforts, and diabetes care and technology.

The ADA also provides support groups, underwrites diabetes summer camps, and lobbies in Congress.

In addition, the ADA uses a portion of its budget for research. It sends out reprints of articles from *Diabetes Forecast* that deal with everything from insulin pumps, to glycemic response, to summer camps and where to find them, to exchanges for fast-food restaurants.

To join the ADA, send $15 for a one-year membership to:

American Diabetes Association
Forecast Membership
PO Box 2043
Mahopac, NY 10541
For information on joining the CDA, write or call:
Canadian Diabetes Association
78 Bond Street
Toronto, Ontario M5B 2J8
(416) 362-4440

For that one-year membership, you receive eight issues of *Diabetes Forecast*, membership in the local ADA affiliate, regular mailings concerning diabetes-related events in your area and local participation in them.

You can find your local ADA chapter by checking your phone book or calling the ADA National Service Center at (800) ADA-DISC.

The Juvenile Diabetes Foundation International has a different emphasis, a singular priority: research to find a cure. We are an almost entirely volunteer organization of parents and diabetics who raise money for research. Over 80 percent of all the money we raise goes directly to research scientists.

In 1972, when JDF was barely two years old, the National Institutes of Health were spending a meager $18 million on diabetes research. A few tireless and dedicated parents played a major role in hearings that led to the enactment of legislation establishing the National Commission on Diabetes. Since then, federal monies for diabetes research have increased to over $190 million—unprecedented growth for a federal health program.

JDF also supplies pamphlets filled with information and a support network of parents, just like you, who won't settle for a lifetime of diabetes for their children.

If you want support for yourself and a cure for your child, join JDF. Check your phone book or call (800) 223-1138.

A call to your local ADA or JDF chapter can help you find

an appropriate doctor. You can ask a doctor you trust for recommendations. You might also see if your public library carries the *Directory of Medical Specialists*. If you need a psychologist, check your local hospital, JDF, or ADA, or consult your diabetes specialist to see if he or she knows of a psychologist who treats children with chronic illness. Ask your sources to recommend someone *they* would trust with *their* child.

NATIONAL DIABETES INFORMATION CLEARINGHOUSE

The National Diabetes Information Clearinghouse was established in 1978 to promote understanding and increase knowledge of the disease among patients, health professionals, and the public. It disseminates information about diabetes to anyone who requests it. It also maintains a computerized file of over 4,000 reference brochures, audiovisual materials, books, articles, and other educational materials. Call or write:

National Diabetes Information Clearinghouse
Box NDIC
Bethesda, MD 20205
(301) 468-2162 or (301) 496-7433

VIDEOTAPES

There are two videotapes available that were recommended by parents I interviewed. One is *Nuts and Bolts of Diabetes*, and it has two parts. One part covers ketoacidosis, and the other discusses low blood sugar. The tapes cost $195 each. The tapes are available on ¾-inch U-Matic or ½-inch Beta or VHS. A preview copy is available for no charge. Call the Audiovisual Department of the University of Colorado at (303) 394-7342 or send a written request to:

Charles Courtier
UCHC
Campus Box A-066
4200 E. 9th Ave.
Denver, CO 80262

The other tape is called *Teacher's Responsibility*. It is geared not only to teachers but also to a wide variety of adults who might be dealing with a diabetic child. It is 20 minutes long and is available from the Montana affiliate of ADA. Call (800) 232-6668 (from inside Montana) or (406) 761-0908. It, too, is available in ¾-inch U-Matic and ½-inch Beta or VHS formats. It costs $295. A preview tape is available for two to three weeks for $30 to anyone who cannot afford to buy it. The tape is copyrighted and cannot be copied.

RECIPE BOOKLETS

The manufacturer of Equal has published three recipe booklets that you might like to have. They are *Equal Delicious Recipes*, *Equal Fruitful Delights*, and *Equal Mocktails*. Send $1 for each or $2.50 for all three booklets to:

Equal Recipes
PO Box 3435
Libertyville, IL 60198

SERVICES FROM DIABETES SUPPLY COMPANIES

There are several sources of diabetic supplies that provide additional services. One is the Sugarfree Center. It is owned by June Biermann and Barbara Toohey, who have written many excellent books, including *The Diabetic's Book* and *The Peripatetic Diabetic*. They are two caring women who are committed to the care and education of diabetic people everywhere. Their center is a full-service facility offering counseling, instruction, and everything you need for diabetes care. They publish a newsletter called *Health-O-Gram* that is filled with information about the latest books and updates on care and attitudes.

Both the Sugarfree Centers are in California, but they have an extensive mail-order list of products and books. To order, call (800) 336-1222 (in California) or (800) 972-2323 (nationwide). If you have questions, you can call (818) 994-1093.

The Diabetic's Answer also provides mail-order service for products and books. On request, it will send you a brochure with articles on diabetes written by doctors. Most of the organization's employees are diabetics. The owner, Erica German, has a three-year-old child with diabetes. Write or call:

The Diabetic's Answer
4962 Grand Ave.
Covina, CA 91724
(818) 915-7773

Penny Saver Drug and Medical Supply is in Denver and offers mail-order service for all diabetes supplies. Call (800) 332-7697 (in Colorado) or (800) 525-7688 (nationwide).

This is only a partial list. I would suggest that you have several mail order companies send their price lists to you so that you can compare prices. You will find other mail order sources listed in ADA's *Diabetes Forecast.*

INSURANCE COMPANIES

The following is a list of insurance companies that have paid or have indicated they will cover pancreas transplants. I provide it as pure information, but also because these companies may provide good coverage for diabetics and their families in other areas:

Aetna Life
Allstate
American Heritage
American Postal Workers Union
Bankers Life of Des Moines
Blue Cross by region: Connecticut, Georgia,
    Massachusetts, Michigan, Nebraska,
    Northeastern Ohio, New Jersey, Oklahoma,
    Pennsylvania, Southern California,
    Tennessee, Wisconsin, Wyoming
Businessmen's Assurance
Connecticut General
Continental Assurance
Continental National America
Equitable Life
Government Employees Hospital Assoc.
Great Southern Life
Hospital Services of Newark
John Alden Insurance
John Hancock
Lewer Insurance/Conaco
Liberty Life
Manitoba Health Plan
Massachusetts Mutual
Metropolitan Life
Minnesota Comprehensive Health
Montana Physicians Service
Mutual of Omaha
National Liberty
New England Mutual
Provident Life
Prudential
Reserve Life
St. Paul Life
Teamsters Union
Trans-Am Occidental
Travelers
United Food and Commercial Workers
Wausau Insurance

Western Life
Western Union
Wisconsin Physicians Services

SUGGESTED READING

I recommend the following books for further reading:

American Diabetes Association. *The American Diabetes Association Family Cookbook Vol. II.* Englewood Cliffs, NJ: Prentice-Hall, Inc., 1984.

Barrett, Andrea. *The Diabetic's Brand Name Food Exchange Handbook.* Philadelphia: Running Press, 1984.

Biermann, June, and Toohey, Barbara. *The Diabetic Book: All Your Questions Answered.* New York: J. P. Tarcher, 1981. (I recommend *anything* written by these authors.)

Brody, Jane. *Jane Brody's Good Food Book.* New York: W. W. Norton & Company, 1985. (Although not for diabetics specifically, this is a great book about good nutrition with hundreds of healthy recipes.)

Cavaiani, Mabel. *The New Diabetic Cookbook.* Chicago: Contemporary Books, Inc., 1984.

Cohen, Sherry Suib, and Ducat, Lee. *Diabetes: A New & Complete Guide to Healthier Living for Parents, Children & Young Adults Who Have Insulin-Dependent Diabetes.* New York: Harper and Row, Publishers, 1983. (This book gets four stars from me.)

Goodman, Joseph I., and Biggers, W. Watts. Paperback ed. *Diabetes Without Fear.* New York: Avon, 1979.

Middleton, Katharine, and Hess, Mary Abbott. *The Art of Cooking for the Diabetic.* Chicago: Contemporary Books, Inc., 1978.

Monk, Arlene, and Franz, Marion J. *Convenience Food Facts*. Minneapolis: International Diabetes Center, 1984. (They publish other booklets you might like to have. Write for a brochure: International Diabetes Center, 5000 West 39th Street, Minneapolis, MN 55416)

Siminerio, Linda, and Betschart, Jean. *Children with Diabetes*. Alexandria, VA: American Diabetes Association, 1986.

MANUFACTURERS

Write to the manufacturers below and ask for informational brochures about their products. There are several gadgets that make life with diabetes a little easier. One is a spring-action lancet holder to help obtain blood for glucose monitoring. There are several styles available: the Autolet, the Auto-Lancet, the Autoclix, and the Penlet. There are also devices that help give injections. One is the Monoject/Inject-O-Matic by Becton-Dickinson. The other is a new model made by Ulster Scientific, Inc., called the Autoject. We're using the Autoject, and Brennan says it has helped cut down the discomfort of injections.

These manufacturers also are sources of educational materials, sample supplies, and funding for educational programs. Most have area representatives who can be located by contacting headquarters.

Ames/Division of Miles Laboratories, Inc.
PO Box 70
Elkhart, IN 46515
(219) 264-8645 or (800) 348-8100

Becton-Dickinson/Consumer Products
365 W. Passaic St.
Rochelle Park, NJ 07662
(201) 848-7100

Boehringer-Mannheim Diagnostics
9115 Hague Rd.
Indianapolis, IN 46250
(317) 845-2000 or (800) 428-5074

Derata Corporation
7380 32nd Ave. N.
Minneapolis, MN 55427
(612) 535-6765 or (800) 328-3074

Diabetes Supplies
8181 N. Stadium Dr.
Houston, TX 77054
(713) 797-1726 or (800) 231-0025

Eli Lilly and Company
Lilly Corporate Center
Indianapolis, IN 46285
(317) 261-2000

Hoechst-Roussel Pharmaceuticals, Inc.
Rte. 202-206 N.
Somerville, NJ 08876
(201) 231-2102

Lifescan, Inc.
2443 Wyandotte St.
Mountain View, CA 94043
(800) 227-8862

Monoject Division of Sherwood Medical
PO Box 14738
St. Louis, MO 63178
(314) 621-7788, (800) 392-7318/Missouri,
or (800) 325-7472

Nordisk
6500 Rock Spring Dr.
Ste. 304
Bethesda, MD 20817
(301) 897-9220

Orange Medical Instruments
3183 Airway Ave.
Suite F
Costa Mesa, CA 92626
(714) 641-5836 or (800) 527-1151

Pfizer Laboratories
Professional Services Dept.
235 E. 42nd St.
New York, NY 10017
(212) 573-2422

Ulster Scientific, Inc.
PO Box 902
Highland, NY 12528
(914) 795-2522, (800) 522-2257/New York,
or (800) 431-8233

13
Research

Up to this point, this book has been geared toward giving you the information that will help you provide the best possible daily care for your diabetic child. Daily blood glucose control is very important, but it is not enough.

Recent studies have indicated that the better the daily control, the greater the possibility of preventing or delaying long-term complications, but there are no guarantees. Diabetes with its complications is still the #3 killer in this country. It is the leading cause of new blindness. I'm not saying this to scare you. That would serve no purpose. I'm saying this to motivate you.

Daily care is very important, but we need something better for our children. We need a cure. I want nothing less than a cure for my son. He used to ask me, "When will my shots be over?" I had to tell him I didn't know.

I want to be able to answer that question. I believe there is every possibility that within five to seven years I will. We are that close. The only thing that stands between us and a cure is money.

Commitment is a powerful tool. It can supply the energy and strength to accomplish anything. I know. I have made a commitment to my son to find a cure for his diabetes. Because of my promise to him, I have dared to accomplish more than I ever dreamed possible.

In a strange way, Brennan's diabetes has been a gift to me. It has expanded my life and broadened my perspective. It has extended my reach and brought seemingly impossible tasks within my grasp.

Is there anything more important than our children? I

can't think of anything. Would you like to be able to cure your child's diabetes? You can.

I have spent the last six years donating my time and talent to the Juvenile Diabetes Foundation. JDF was founded 15 years ago by Lee Ducat and a handful of other mothers. They wanted to know what was being done to find a cure for their children. They found that there was very little research. They decided that wasn't good enough. They formed a foundation of volunteers, JDF, that as of today has given more money to diabetes research than any organization in the world, other than the U.S. government. JDF is an almost entirely volunteer group of parents who won't take no for an answer. We are the militants, the movers and shakers. Because of our perseverance, there is more emphasis today on diabetes and research than ever before. We have made an enormous difference—and our children will reap the benefits.

I have been shocked and frustrated to hear of parents who say they are too busy to join JDF. I can't imagine anything that could take priority over our children's health. In addition to helping to find a cure, JDF puts us in touch with each other, parents and children who now know we're not alone.

The original intent of this chapter was to give you a general idea of the advances in diabetes research in recent years. As I gathered information, it became apparent to me that the research being done demanded a more thorough reporting. The result here is a detailed, often technical explanation of the current state of Type I diabetes research. I offer it as encouragement, motivation, and hope for the future.

Only a small percentage of parents whose children are affected by diabetes are actively involved in fundraising to find a cure. One eminent researcher, Dr. Paul Lacy, recently remarked that 90% of what we know about diabetes has been learned in the last ten years. Think what progress we could make if everyone affected joined the fight to end diabetes. Think what the next ten years could bring.

CAUSES

In order to appreciate the complexity of the answers researchers are seeking, we need to understand the causes of diabetes and the questions that are raised.

Type I diabetes (also called juvenile diabetes) occurs when the beta-cells in the pancreas are destroyed. The beta cells produce insulin, a hormone that is essential for metabolism and life. Researchers have identified three potential causes of this destruction. They seem to involve a genetic factor, the immune system, and a triggering mechanism.

Type I diabetes is a disease of genetic susceptibility. That means your child was born with a genetic background that makes him prone to get diabetes. Not everyone with this genetic predisposition gets the disease, but you cannot get it if the genetic susceptibility is not present. This genetic defect appears to be in the genes that control the body's ability to recognize its own tissue as friend or foe.

The immune system is like a hit squad that seeks out intruders and destroys them. In Type I diabetes, the body is no longer able to recognize the beta cells as part of itself. It is fooled into identifying the beta cells as foreign invaders. Various parts of the immune system that are actually designed to prevent infection then target the cells and produce antibodies to destroy them. These antibodies to insulin-producing cells may be found in some diabetics months, even years, before the actual symptoms of diabetes begin. The antibodies probably knock off the beta cells a little at a time.

The infection (or whatever) that causes the final destruction acts as a kind of triggering mechanism. Stress and viruses have been implicated as possible causes. For example, diagnoses of diabetes rise during the flu season. Maybe the flu virus exacerbates the condition by leaving the body susceptible, or maybe the flu virus acts as the trigger. It may someday be possible to alter a person's genetic susceptibility to diabetes, but that's a long shot and will take years more research.

However, scientists are already experimenting with drugs to try to turn off the immune system so that it won't destroy the beta cells in the pancreas, which produce insulin. They have found ways to intervene in the destruction of beta cells in animals. Human trials are being conducted right now. The problem is that the drugs being used, cyclosporin and prednisone, have serious side effects and are not practical for long-term use. They have shown that intervention is possible because when patients began using these drugs soon after diagnosis, they went into a honeymoon phase when no insulin was required. However, it lasted only as long as they took the drugs. The goal now is to find safer drugs.

Scientists are also trying to identify the mechanisms that cause the final destruction of the beta cells. If they can, they'll be able to protect people with diabetes from them. For example, if specific viruses are found to trigger the immune system, then perhaps a vaccine could be developed.

TREATMENT AND CURE

Our children produce little or no insulin of their own. Externally produced insulin must be delivered into the body. Since insulin was discovered in 1921, the traditional treatment for Type I diabetes has been one or more injections of insulin a day. A nondiabetic person's pancreas produces only as much insulin as is needed to allow glucose to be converted into energy. Taking one or two injections a day does not mimic this precise process. As a result, diabetics may be subjected to wide fluctuations in blood sugar levels.

In addition, there is evidence that both too much or too little insulin itself may lead to complications. One of the objectives of research is to find better ways to deliver insulin into a body not producing its own. Several new techniques have been developed.

The insulin pump is a device that infuses insulin into the body at a preprogrammed rate throughout the day, with the patient programming doses for each meal. The newest models are about the size of a mini-calculator. Researchers are attempting to miniaturize the pumps even further, so that they can be implanted within the body. In addition, scientists are attempting to develop a small glucose sensor that could automatically measure blood sugar levels. If such a sensor could be developed and attached to an insulin pump, it could function as an implantable artificial pancreas.

Another possible method of insulin delivery is the nasal spray. Scientists have ascertained that the nasal membranes may be a good spot for insulin to be administered. The problems have been increasing the absorption from the nose into the bloodstream and developing ways to prevent irritation of the nasal passages. Researchers are now developing agents which, when mixed with insulin, allow the nose to be used. The nasal spray uses regular insulin only. While a nasal insulin spray will never completely eliminate the need for injections, it is hoped that, in the future, people with diabetes will be able to increase the number of times they take insulin by taking some injections and a few sprays daily. That way, they could more closely approximate the body's response to rises in blood sugar. It is hoped that the nasal spray will be available in a few years.

Those of us who work closely with JDF and the researchers feel that the most exciting possibilities lie in beta cell transplants. Beta cell transplants have cured diabetes in some animals, and human trials have begun. One major stumbling block is that we're not sure that the body won't seek out these cells and destroy them as it did the original beta cells. Scientists must be able to prevent the immune system's destructive process.

A number of techniques are being tried to solve this problem. Some researchers are developing drugs that can prevent rejection. Others are attempting to microencapsulate the cells to prevent rejection. This is done by wrapping the cell in a porous, plastic-type material. The pores are large enough to let the insulin out but too small to allow the immune system in to destroy the beta cells. This has worked in dogs for up to two years.

Another technique is to culture the cells in certain chemicals at a particular temperature. Proteins on the surface of the cells help the body identify the cells as foreign. These proteins are called antigens. The antigens act as stimulators and send the message to the immune system that the tissue is foreign. The culturing of the beta cells either silences or destroys the antigens (we're not sure which). When they're transplanted, they are not identified as foreign and, hence, are not attacked. This technique has worked in animals and is now being researched using human cells.

The question of where to put the beta cells is not settled. Scientists don't want to put them into the pancreas because it is too complicated an organ and too risky. They've succeeded in animals by injecting the cells into the spleen, the portal vein (to the liver), the abdominal cavity, and under the kidney capsule.

Two other problems also presented themselves. One is tissue procurement. Beta cells are difficult to obtain because there is an insufficient supply of donor pancreases. Even when a pancreas does become available, it is difficult to separate the insulin producing cells from the rest of the organ.

The other difficulty is tissue storage. After the cells have been harvested, but prior to transplantation, the beta cells must be properly stored to prevent spoilage. Scientists are working on a way to freeze the cells at very low temperatures so that they can store them indefinitely. This has also worked in animal research.

In preparing this chapter, I spoke with several prominent researchers. Two of them are leading the way in the area of beta cell transplants. Dr. Kevin Lafferty and Dr. Paul Lacy are working on two different approaches to beta cell transplants that are fascinating and very promising.

Dr. Kevin Lafferty is working on transplanting undifferentiated islet tissue. To put it simply, he is transplanting the seeds from which the beta cells grow. In the first trials, he transplanted the cells into five patients' stomachs. (These are people who were undergoing kidney transplants at the same time.) It didn't work. The question was why? Were there not enough cells? Didn't they grow? Were they in the wrong position? Or did the body try to destroy them again?

In the new series of experiments Dr. Lafferty is doing, he is implanting the cells into the kidney capsule (the casing of the kidney). He is able to take a tissue sample of the implanted cells right through the skin, without surgery. The tissue sample has provided many answers.

Three to four months after implantation, the tissue is alive, new blood vessels are forming, and the islet seeds are becoming mature beta cells that contain insulin. Dr. Lafferty says, "I am definitely optimistic and feel we've taken the first step toward the ultimate clinical application of this technology." He also told me that beta cell transplants being available in five to seven years as a treatment/cure is within the realm of possibility.

Dr. Paul Lacy is working on transplanting mature human islet cells. (Islet cells contain beta cells and other naturally occurring cells that produce additional important hormones.) At first, he put the cells, which he described as fairly "rough," into the spleen. They functioned for one to two months. These initial trials were encouraging. He has now developed a highly purified sample of the islet cells and is inserting them into the liver. He has also developed a process to preserve the islets outside the body. He can test their function to be sure they are alive and producing hormones, which could not be done previously.

Dr. Lacy is "extremely encouraged by the findings thus far. The critical studies are yet to come, but it could have been a case when *nothing* worked and we would have been back to the bench for 10 years!"

Pancreas transplants have been taking place since 1966. The first long-term successes were accomplished with the grafts done in 1978. As of today, 830 pancreas transplants have been done. Of the ones done since 1983, 45% are functioning. Most of these transplants were done in conjunction with a kidney transplant. This type of procedure is a major surgery and requires that immuno-suppressive drugs be taken indefinitely. The drugs are given at a low dose, but it still means a trade-off. The patient trades the complications of diabetes for the complications of immunosuppressive drugs.

Currently, candidates for transplant must be at least 18 years old and display signs of complications. The transplant is considered a therapeutic procedure and is covered by quite a few insurers (in "Resources," see index). It is an expensive surgery. Pancreas transplant programs are now under way at the Universities of Minnesota, Wisconsin, Iowa, and Michigan. Dr. David Sutherland at the University of Minnesota feels that, if enough organs could be obtained, the pancreas transplant would be as common as the kidney transplant (which numbers 6,000 a year).

There's another idea that is revolutionary and considered a long shot, but which is fascinating. It would be to teach another cell to do the job of the beta cell. As far-fetched as it sounds, conceptually it's very much like the procedure for producing human insulin.

Human insulin is synthesized by using recombinant DNA technology. It eliminates dependence on animals and their pancreas glands as the sole source of insulin. It is highly purified and helps reduce allergic reactions and the loss of subcutaneous tissue at the injection sites. It is the first important medical product of genetic engineering to be used by a large segment of the public. Check with your child's doctor to see if your child should be using synthesized human insulin.

GET INVOLVED *NOW*

As you can see, diabetes is a tremendously complicated disease. We are still a long way from having all the answers, but we wouldn't have any answers if it weren't for the researchers who have been working for the last 15 to 20 years.

These researchers are now using many of their findings on humans. Human trials are enormously expensive. As I said, the only thing that stands between our children and a cure is money. Biomedical research is greatly threatened by recent federal budget cuts. In addition, animal rights groups are trying to bring an end to all animal research. Parents of children with chronic illness understand their child's life will be greatly affected by the quality of research and the development of new answers.

There is no time to lose. If every parent of a diabetic child were to join us now and actively work for a cure, we could have one in maybe five years. Help me save my son's eyesight, his kidneys, the quality of his health and life. I will do the same for your child.

Master List of Recipes

APPETIZERS

BEVERAGES

SOUPS

BREADS AND CEREALS

MAIN COURSES

MEAT

BEEF AND VEAL

LAMB

Baked Lamb Chops,
   page 253
Greek Lamb Chops,
   page 251

Lovely Lamb Stew,
   page 252

PORK

Orange Pork Chops with
   Rice, *page 254*

POULTRY

BBQ Chicken, *page 219*
Brunswick Stew, *page 224*
Chicken Cacciatore,
   page 215
Chicken Cordon Bleu,
   page 223
Chicken Pizzaiola,
   page 222
Chicken and Vegetable
   Stir-Fry, *page 214*
Foiled Chicken, *page 217*
Lemon Chicken, *page 213*
Lemon Chicken with
   Bulgur, *page 216*

Orange Chicken, *page 218*
Oven-Fried Chicken,
   page 220
Peanut Butter Chicken,
   page 221
Roast Stuffed Turkey,
   page 226
Turkey Burgers, *page 229*
Turkey Chili, *page 142*
Turkey Loaf, *page 225*
Turkey Tetrazzini,
   page 230

FISH

Foiled Fish Fillets,
   page 235
Oven Fish Fillets,
   page 236
Oven "French-Fried"
   Scallops, *page 233*

Salmon Croquettes,
   page 236
Saucy Scallops, *page 234*
Seafood Stew, *page 232*

PASTA SALADS, SANDWICHES, VEGETARIAN DISHES

Baked Macaroni and
   Cheese, *page 140*
Cheese Blintzes, *page 96*
Chili Deluxe with
   Vegetables, *page 143*

Chinese Chicken Salad,
   page 210
Eggs Benedict, *page 86*
Fast Spaghetti Sauce with
   Spaghetti Squash, *page 208*

VEGETABLES
STARCHY

NONSTARCHY

SIDE DISHES AND SALADS

SAUCES, DRESSINGS, AND CONDIMENTS

SWEET TREATS AND DESSERTS

Index

ADA (American Diabetes
    Association), 353–55
Adolescence, diabetes control,
    313–15
Adolescence, stages of, 312
Alcohol consumption, effect
    on diabetics, 344–45
Alcohol consumption and
    insulin reaction, 345
All-American cranberry
    sauce, 293
Ambrosia, 81
Apple(s)
    -cran crisp, 296
    crunch, 173
    pancake, baked, 93
    salad, 167
    spice oatmeal, 83
    spiced baked, 82
    squash with, 267
Applesauce, 114
    bran squares, 180
    muffins, 106
Appliances, types of, 50
Aspartame in diet, 10–11
Associations (ADA, JDA, etc.)
    for diabetics, 353–55

Bacon in diet, 70
Baked
    apple pancake 93

beans, 141
custard, 168
lamb chops, 253
macaroni and cheese, 140
spinach, 275
Baking dishes, types of, 48
Baking powder, 66
Banana(s)
    bread, 101
    cream pie, quick, 176–77
    frozen, 163
    shake, 77
    and sweet potatoes, 264
BBQ chicken, 219
Bean(s)
    baked, 141
    dip, 157
    navy, soup, 125
    -potato patties, 260–61
    red, and rice, 256
Beef
    flank steak, Oriental, 241
    pot roast, 243
    and snow peas, 242
    stew, superb oven, 246
    Swiss steak, 245
    and tomato stir-fry, 240
    -vegetable soup, 130
Beef, ground
    chili deluxe, 143
    meat and vegetable loaf, 244

sautéed, 272
tart red, 271
Cacciatore chicken, 215
Cake, carrot snack, 181
Cake, vanilla cheesecake,
  182–83
Camping, special meals for,
  51–53
Carbohydrates, complex. *See
  also* Fiber
  for breakfast, 71
  in diet, 16–19
Carrot(s)
  -acorn squash, 265
  fruit spiced, 273
  and raisin salad, 166
  snack cake, 181
Cauliflower or broccoli
  parmesan, 269
CDA (Canadian Diabetes
  Association), 353–54
Cereal, apple spice oatmeal,
  83
Cereals, breakfast choices,
  71–72
Cheese. *See also* Cottage
  cheese
  blintzes, 96
  raisin toast, 90
Cheesecake, vanilla, 182–83
Cherry pie, 175
Chicken. *See also* Turkey
  about cooking, 7
  BBQ, 219
  Brunswick stew, 224
  cacciatore, 215
  Cordon Bleu, 223
  foiled, 217
  lemon, 213
  lemon with bulgur, 216
  orange, 218

oven-fried, 220
peanut butter, 221
pizzaiola, 222
salad, Chinese, 210–11
sandwich, pita pockets,
  137
and vegetable stir-fry, 214
Childhood development,
  303–4, 308–9, 312
Chili deluxe with vegetables,
  143
Chili, turkey, 142
Chinese chicken salad,
  210–11
Chinese vegetables, 281
Chocolate
  chip cookies, 171
  delight, 291
  sauce, 292
  shake, 154
Cholesterol
  blood, 6
  in fats, 5
  foods containing, 6
Chowder, clam, Manhattan,
  128
Chowder, corn, 129
Cinnamon toast, 91
Clam chowder, Manhattan,
  128
Clam sauce, red, linguine
  with, 197
Cocoa mix, homemade, 79
Coleslaw, 146
Coleslaw, special fruited, 147
Complex carbohydrates. *See*
  Carbohydrates
Convulsions, 338–39
Cookies
  applesauce bran squares,
  180

brownies, "wholesome,"
    128
chocolate chip, 171
oatmeal, 174
peanut butter, 170
Cordon Bleu chicken, 223
Corn chowder, 129
Corn pudding, 266
Cornbread, Gloria's, 99
Cottage cheese orange
    muffins, 108
Cracked wheat. See Bulgur
Cran-apple crisp, 296
Cranberry
    cran-apple crisp, 296
    mold, 295
    relish, 294
    sauce, all-American, 293
Creamy vinaigrette, 287
Crêpes, bran, 97
Cucumber salad, 274
Custard, baked, 168

Dairy products, place in diet,
    7-8
"Dawn phenomenon,"
    330-31
Dessert, 290-97. *See also*
    Name of fruit; Pies; etc.
    chocolate delight, 291
    chocolate sauce, 292
    custard, baked, 168
    lemon snow pudding, 290
    rice pudding, Brennan's,
        169
    sherbert, orange, 164-65
    sherbert, pineapple, 165
Devilish eggs, 161
Diabetes
    advice to parents about,
        316-19

and alcohol consumption,
    344-45
associations, 353
behavior problems, 306-7
blood sugar control, 324,
    330-31
blood sugar testing, 307,
    311
causes of, 365-66
coma, diabetic, 333
control during adolescence,
    313-16
control during childhood,
    309-11
control during illness,
    331-34
control in infants and
    toddlers, 304-8
daily care, importance of,
    363
emergency, how to handle,
    343
explaining to children, 304
family support, 4, 316-17
fat and cholesterol, role of, 5
genetic predisposition,
    365-66
health insurance for,
    345-51, 357-59
and the immune system,
    365-68
information, getting
    correct, 326-27, 29
insulin reactions, 307-8,
    335-39
management, 65
medical care for, 322-24
medical products suppliers,
    361-62
psychological adjustments,
    301-2

Fatty acids, 6; Omega-3 long
   chain, 5–6
Fiber
   and complex carbohydrates
      in diet, 16–19
   incorporation in diet
      (example), 18
   water-soluble, 16
Fish. *See also* Name of fish;
      Seafood
   in diet, 8
   fillets, foiled, 235
   fillets, oven, 236
   low cholesterol of, 8
   salmon croquettes, 236–37
   saturated fat in, 5
   sauce, mustard, 237
Flank steak, Oriental, 241
Flounder, oven fish fillets,
   236
Flour, whole wheat, 17
Flours and grains, in pantry,
   43–44
Foiled chicken, 217
Foiled fish fillets, 235
Food exchanges, 21–37
"French-fried," oven, scallops,
   233
"French fries," oven, 259
French toast, 92
Fresh blueberry sauce, 113
Fresh peach pie, 178
Frozen banana, 163
Frozen fruit treats, 164
Fructose in diet, 12–13
Fruit(s). *See also* Name of
      fruit
   about using, 66–67
   berry yogurt, 80
   dip, peanut, 158
   exchanges in diet, 26–27

high in fiber, 17
spiced carrots, 273
treats, frozen, 164
Fruited coleslaw, special, 147

Garlic, about using, 67
German potato salad, 145
Gloria's cornbread, 99
Gloria's spaghetti sauce,
   206–7; with meat, 207
Glucagon, 331–32, 338
Glucose, 335–36. *See also*
   Blood sugar
Glucose, blood, monitoring,
   323
Glycemic index, 19–20
Glycosolated hemoglobin, 340
Graham cracker crust, 177
Grain(s). *See also* Whole
      grains
   bread, high-protein, three-
      grain, 102–3
   bread, Irish soda whole
      grain, 104
   and flours, in pantry,
      43–44
Granola, commercial, 71
Granola, stovetop, 84
Grape soda, 154
Gravy from meat drippings,
   289
Greek lamb chops, 251
Greek lemon soup, 135

Hamburgers. *See* Turkey
      burgers
Hash brown turnips, 280
Health insurance for
      diabetics, 345–50
Health maintenance
      organizations (HMOs), 350